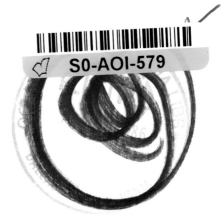

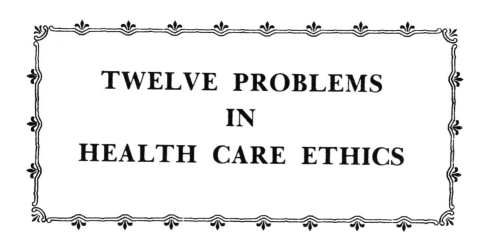

TWELVE PROBLEMS
IN
HEALTH CARE ETHICS

STUDIES IN HEALTH AND HUMAN SERVICES

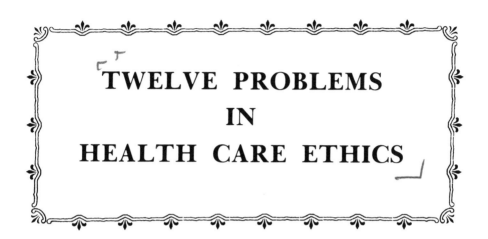

TWELVE PROBLEMS IN
HEALTH CARE ETHICS

Thomas A. Shannon, Ph.D.

Studies in Health and Human Services
Volume Two

The Edwin Mellen Press
New York and Toronto

Library of Congress Cataloging In Publication Data

Shannon, Thomas Anthony, 1940-
   Twelve problems in health care ethics.

   (Studies in health and human services ; vol. 2)
   1. Medical ethics--Addresses, essays, lectures.
2. Abortion--Government policy--United States--
Addresses, essays, lectures. I. Title. II. Series:
Studies in health and human services ; v. 2.
R725.5.S53 1985   174'.2   84-22654
ISBN 0-88946-127-9

Studies in Health and Human Services
Series ISBN 0-88946-126-0

The Edwin Mellen Press
P.O. Box 450
Lewiston, New York 14092

Printed in the United States of America

To my wife Cathy
who has made my life flourish.

CONTENTS

TWELVE PROBLEMS
IN
HEALTH CARE ETHICS

ABORTION

A Review of Ethical Aspects of Public Policy

The purpose of this paper is to review and analyze several issues related to the debate about public policy on abortion. What I hope to do in this article is review some of the ethical and political issues raised in abortion, describe some aspects of abortion policy in America, identify ethical problems raised by some of the policy questions, and then discuss some of the ethical issues involved in these policy debates. What I hope to accomplish by this is to indicate some fundamental problems in the debate and hope that we can focus on some of the more substantive issues behind the debate.

1. A Review of Policy and Incidence of Abortion.

According to Christopher Tietze[1] as of late 1980, about 9% of the world's population lived in countries where abortion was prohibited without exception and about 19% of the world's population lived in countries where it was permitted only to save the life of a pregnant woman. Fewer than 10% live in countries where statutes authorize abortions on broader medical grounds, i.e., averting a threat to a woman's health rather than only to her life, and occasionally for eugenic or fetal indications. About 24% of the world's population were able to take into account social factors such as income, housing, marital status in evaluating a woman's health. About 38% of the population live in countries which allow abortion on request without specifying a reason and this is generally limited to the first trimester of pregnancy.

These policies also have a wide range of applicability. A policy authorizing abortion to avert a threat to a pregnant woman's health could be defined narrowly or broadly. Social indications for abortion may similarly be defined. Many statutes may not be strictly enforced and, in any event, whatever statutes there are rely upon the cooperation of health care providers and delivery systems. Consequently, even though a particular country may have a liberal abortion policy which is guaranteed by statute, that does not necessarily mean that the procedure is actually available to any woman who wants an abortion.

Within the last 15 years, many countries have liberalized their abortion laws; 4 countries in Eastern Europe adopted more restrictive legislation and 3 countries liberalized their policies and then made them more restrictive.

The reasons used by proponents of less restrictive abortion legislation are summarized as follows: consideration of public health, especially the morbidity and mortality associated with illegal abortion; social justice, allowing poor women to have equal access to abortion; women's rights, including the right to control their own bodies. Only a few countries - Singapore, Indonesia, and China - have used the explicit motivation of curbing population growth in the interest of economic and social development as a reason for adopting nonrestrictive abortion policies. Ironically, many countries which permit abortions either at the request of the woman or on broadly interpreted social indications have low birth rates and some of these countries are now actively pursuing pronatalist population policies.[2]

Although highly speculative, the number of abortions internationally has been estimated at around 55,000,000

which would correspond to an abortion rate of around 70
per 1,000 women of abortion age and an abortion ratio of
300 per 1,000 known pregnancies.

The differences in abortion rates in the United
States between whites and blacks are interesting.
Between 1963 and 1965 among whites, the abortion rate was
.19 per 1,000 and from 1966 to 1968 it was .20 per 1,000.
During those same years it was .17 and .29 for blacks
respectively.   In 1978 the abortion rate for whites was
22.7 and 60.4 per 1,000 for blacks.[3]

2.   A Review of Policies on Abortion in the United
      States

In his book, Mohr traces the history of why in 1800
there were virtually no abortion policies, in 1900 every
state had an antiabortion law.   While not wanting to
rehearse all of the salient elements in Mohr's book,
there are a few issues with respect to public policy and
abortion that I want to emphasize.

Mohr identifies several motives why the early
abortion legislation came into being.   The first motive
focused on preventing the mother's death through the use
of an abortifacient.[4]   These laws, as Mohr notes, were
primarily poison control measures focusing not so much on
the fetus as on the health status of the mother and the
safety of the procedure that was used.   These laws also
had the effect of reinforcing the traditional norm of
"quickening" as the dividing line between abortions which
were not governed by statutes and those which were.   The
other two motives Mohr says contributed to the increase
in abortion laws, especially coming to a climax point at
the end of the nineteenth century, have to do with changes
in the perception of who was receiving an abortion and
who was providing the procedure.   There was a growing
fear that since first generation American

women were now receiving abortions at high rates, the
WASP population might be outnumbered by the immigrants.
This perception was related to the developing nativist
movement and consequently statutes were enacted to
restrict abortion, intending not the protection of the
fetus, but the protection of the status and power of
the established classes. Parallel to this was the growing professionalization of   medicine. Physicians
were interested both in developing and tightening their
own standards of practice and in eliminating from
medicine those described as quacks. Physicians lobbied
against abortion to eliminate from the profession individuals who would not abide by its rules and as a
means of controlling the standards of the members of
the profession itself. The medical profession was also
further able to control abortion by helping define
medical conditions under which abortion might be appropriate and by providing competent individuals to
perform the procedure. Thus, by the end of the nineteenth century, abortion legislation was present in
all of the states and was contrary to the earlier experience of the country in which abortion was possible
for those who wanted it. Again the primary intent of
this legislation was the protection of the mother and
the enhancement of the social status of two different
groups within society: the establishment and physicians.

          Mohr also describes the pressures that led to
the reevaluation of these antiabortion statutes in our
own time which led to the Roe V. Wade decision in
1972.[5] These pressures are: 1) the fear of overpopu-
lation; 2) a growing concern for the quality of life
of the fetus as opposed to the mere preservation of
life; 3) the development of the Women's Rights Movement with its emphasis on a woman's right to control

her body; 4) the growing safety of abortion done under
appropriate medical conditions; 5) the fact that women
were getting abortions anyway in spite of restrictive
legislation. One could also add to this list the movement of several states to relax their own abortion
legislation. Ultimately this led to the testing of restrictive state statutes in the Supreme Court.

What is important from this survey is that
abortion legislation was developed primarily out of a
variety of social issues that were not directly or quite
possibly even indirectly related to concern for the
fetus. The older use of the term quickening and its
contemporary analogue of viability, served as a touch-
stone for the limits of abortion. That is, in the early
nineteenth century, abortion was not considered problematic morally or medically until the point of quickening. In the view of many individuals, a similar argument
is being made today from at least a medical, if not a
moral point of view. And, in fact, as Mohr indicates,
the Roe decision is based somewhat upon this older
traditional view within American society: abortions
before quickening or viability are not problematic.
But again what I think Mohr focuses on is the social
context for the development of abortion legislation and
its repeal. Abortion statutes - whether pro or con -
were based upon neither the sanctity of life of the fetus
or a disregard of it, but rather upon other social
issues and concerns.

Another important review of abortion policies
comes from a recent article by Tatalovich and Daynes,
entitled, "The Trauma of Abortion Politics."[6] These
authors indicate three significant periods in the history of the policy debate. First, in the early 60's
the basic issue was the building of a consensus toward

abortion reform which focused primarily on the availability of therapeutic abortion. The authors note
that the pro-abortion advocates shared similar assumptions, made similar arguments and held common objectives
with the abortion opponents. These proponents assumed,
based on the American Law Institute's recommendations,
that abortion should be permitted only to a limited
number of women and that it should be performed for
therapeutic reasons. This position defines abortion
primarily in medical terms, not moral ones. The abortion reformers were not making any radical claims.
All of the abortion statutes in effect permitted therapeutic abortions when the mother's life was in danger.
Some states allowed abortion when the mother's health
was threatened. What the reformers were arguing for
was an incremental change in the abortion laws allowing this more expanded exception. And at that point
in time approximately 80% of the general population
favored some abortion reform, and while this support
came from both Catholics and Protestants, Catholics did
not support the reform at the same level that the Protestants did.

        A second critical period that the authors iden-
tify is 1969 to 1970 which was shaped by three inter-
related developments. First, the pro-abortionists
shifted towards repeal of all abortion laws as opposed
to therapeutic reform. Second, opposition to abortion
began to focus on opposition to any change, thereby
opposing not only the new movement towards total repeal of abortion laws, but even the incremental changes
that were desired earlier. Third, the proponents of
abortion began to shift their strategy to the use of
the judiciary to achieve reform rather than expend their
limited resources on attempts to change legislation

state by state. This strategy culminated in Roe which
had a winner take all dimension. This court decision
made it difficult for any compromise posture to be taken
and helped change the nature of the debate. Interest-
ingly enough the authors point out that there were ample
court precedents on either side of the issue and that
the court was not inherently locked into a pro-abortion
decision. But had the court come out the other way,
there still would have been a public policy debate, with
the sides reversed. A major problem is not so much the
court's decision, as the winner take all nature of the
decision which has in effect polarized the debate.

The third issue has to do with this polarization
of perceptions on abortion as well as strategies to
achieve the ends of the antiabortion groups. One of
the by-products of this polarization has been the
legislative maneuverings of the antiabortion group.
Picking up their cues for strategies for reform from
the pro-abortion groups, the antiabortion groups have
gone them one better and chosen to go neither the state
legislative route nor the route of the judiciary but
rather are attempting to circumvent the entire judicial system by having certain kinds of legislation
declared off limits from federal judicial review. The
antiabortion people recognize that state by state cam-
paigns will be costly and time consuming; they realize
that a constitutional amendment may be very difficult
to achieve. One effective strategy is to circumvent
these processes by having Congress declare certain
forms of legislation off limits to judicial review.
They are also attempting to devise federal legislation
to restrict public monies for abortion to as few cases
as possible so that those who wish abortions must pay
for them themselves. Two important moves here have

been legislation introduced to define life as beginning at conception - thus ensuring a fetus constitutional rights, making abortion illegal, and raising
constitutional problems regarding certain forms of con-
traception - and the Hatch amendment, recently passed
by the Senate Judiciary Subcommittee, which states the
right to an abortion is not secured by the Constitution
and that the states and Congress shall have power to
restrict and prohibit abortions. This amendment gives
a state law precedence if it is more restrictive than
federal legislation. Thus the third major phase of the
debate that these authors identify consists of a conflict
at a very high and intense level among groups who are
violently pro or con abortion, while simultaneously
denying to legislatures the ability to make compromise
moves. By focusing on an either/or position, consensus
is more difficult to achieve and consequently no policy
is able to gain legitimacy. Our current debate is
characterized by polarization and a move from a debate
of the issues to personal confrontations in which parties
are perceived to be liberal or conservative with respect
to how they perceive this particular issue.

3.   Opinions on Abortion.

        One of the issues that is important in develop-
ing a public policy is to insure some sense of legitimacy
of this policy by rooting it in the beliefs of the
citizenry so that the policy at least to some degree will
be acceptable and workable. I am not arguing that the
morality of abortion will be settled or determined by
poll taking; I do think it is important, with respect
to proposing and implementing policy, to attend to perceptions about abortion and to determine if there are
possible connections between the pro and con abortion
groups that might help facilitate some kind of compromise
to enable a policy to be developed.

We need to examine first what reasons for abortion
people find persuasive. One important finding is that
there is an average approval of 67% for six specific reasons for abortion: a woman's health is seriously endangered by the pregnancy; becoming pregnant as a result of
rape; a strong chance of a serious defect in the baby; the
family has a low income and cannot afford anymore children;
the woman is pregnant and does not want to marry the man;
the woman is married and does not want anymore children.[7]
The last three reasons are known as the "soft" reasons
for abortion and there is no solid social consensus on
these three. The average consensus for the first three
reasons, the "hard" reasons, averages about 85%, whereas
it is about 50% for the soft reasons. There is clearly
strong social consensus around the broadened concept of a
therapeutic abortion. There is less, but slightly increasing, support for the more social or personal reasons for
wanting an abortion. It is also important to note that
the average approval has changed only four percentage
points since 1972. There was a jump of twenty-two points
between 1965 and 1972. But there has been a remarkable
stability in the approval rate since 1972.[8]

With respect to the profiles of those engaged in
the debate, there are some interesting correlations. First,
two relevant differences between those who are pro and con
abortion is that those who are antiabortion tend to feel
that obedience is more important and that curiosity during
child development is less important than do those who are
in favor of abortion. Second, a finding which should sur-
prise no one, the higher a person's social status, the
greater is their tendency to approve abortion. In fact
one study indicated that a formal education is the best
predictor of abortion attitudes. Third, the more one dis-
approves of activities such as premarital sex, extramari-
tal sex, and homosexuality, the less one favors abortion.

Fourth, differences between Protestants and Catholics with respect to favoring or not favoring abortion increase in proportion to the degree of education that the individual has had. Finally, for both Protestants and Catholics approval of abortion decreases as religiosity indexes increase, with the notable exception of Episcopalians who are more likely to approve of abortion the more religious they are. What is significantly interesting and important in one study was the allegation that the Protestant-Catholic difference accounts for only about 1% of the variation in abortion attitudes over the years. This leads to the interesting hypothesis that the religious differences are not the critical differences in the abortion debate and that to cast the debate in terms of religious preference is both mistaken and particularly counterproductive for policy debates. These studies would indicate that the critical variables are those beyond religion and having to do with feelings about child rearing, social practices, education, and class.[9]

A study of differences between members of the National Abortion Rights Action League (NARAL) and the National Right to Life Committee (NRLC) showed some interesting differences with respect to what the membership of each organization felt about abortion.[10] These findings are of particular importance for policy making. More than 95% of NARAL members and fewer than 5% of NRLC members approve of legal abortion when there is a strong chance of a serious defect in the baby, when the woman is married and wants no more children, when a women's husband will not consent to an abortion and when an unmarried woman wants to have an abortion. These data are

not surprising, especially insofar as they refer to the
soft reasons for abortion. However, it's interesting
that 73% of NRLC members favor making abortion available
to women whose life is endangered by continuation of the
pregnancy. Also 15% of NRLC members approve of abortion
if the pregnant woman's physical health is seriously endangered by carrying the pregnancy to term and 7% to 8%
favor legal abortion if pregnancy is the result of rape
or incest. These data indicate that members of the NRLC
do not present as monolithic and absolutistic position
on abortion as might be assumed. While the policy that
could be based on such feelings may not be acceptable
to all, nonetheless it does indicate that there are
possibilities for some movement. Compromise, of course,
will be called for.

Another relevant factor revealed by this survey
indicates that NRLC activists are not only generally
more conservative on moral issues but are also likely
to describe themselves as conservatives, as Republicans,
and to oppose government action to reduce income differences between rich and poor. As important as those
differences are, the NRLC members are much more likely
than NARAL members to give priority to their views on
abortion over their views on social issues. Eighty-
four percent of NRLC members as opposed to 47% of NARAL
members say that abortion is so important that they would
refuse to support a candidate whose position on abortion
was unacceptable. This may mean that in elections or
in debates of public policy, all other things being
equal, there may be a strategic advantage to having a
group which has the higher percentage of single issue
voters on its side.

An interesting perspective is revealed on the
single-mindedness of many of the right to life movement
by another analysis of activists in the prolife movement.[11] Kelley identified some general reasons why they
were concerned for only one issue. First, abortion stops
a human life and is, therefore, a unique issue. Second,
a single issue focus protects the right to life movement
from being absorbed or manipulated by any political
party. Third, the passage of a human life amendment to
the Constitution requires a political coalition of
people with different ideologies and, therefore, stra-
tegically they wish to avoid being perceived as members
of any other group. There seems to be a recognition
that the alliance present in the prolife movement is
very tenuous and that it might not be able to stand the
strain of having to deal with social problems that may
not be perceived as having the same importance or solution, e.g., nuclear war or social welfare programs.

It would be interesting to know how the structure
and impact of the prolife movement will be affected by
the interior tensions that are present, at least with
respect to differences in the kinds of approvals of
abortion that are tolerated by some members. The monolithic unity of the prolife movement may be a perception,
not a reality. One could assume that much of the energy
of the prolife movement needs to be spent in making sure
that potentially disruptive issues do not enter into
the dialogue and that no relationship between the ethical values surrounding the evaluation of abortion and
other social issues be made, i.e., extending a prolife
stance to evaluate nuclear war. One could make a
reasonable case that such a position will continue to
become more and more difficult as time goes on and that
members of prolife groups will have to make more and

more difficult choices with respect to the supporting
of political candidates, especially when these candidates
present viewpoints on a variety of issues that may, in
fact, appeal to different populations within the prolife
movement.

4.   Ethical Issues and the Setting of Policy

        Kelman and Warwick identify two important aspects
of social intervention and the setting of public policy
that can raise major ethical issues.[12] First are the
four aspects of the policy intervention that inherently
raise ethical issues. These include:

        1)   the choice of goals to which the change effort
             is directed

        2)   the definition of the target of the change

        3)   the choice of means used to implement the
             intervention

        4)   the assessment of the consequences of this
             intervention.

        Each of these particular steps raises a variety
of value issues, at least in terms of which values will
be sacrificed for others and what kind of an intervention will maximize the implementation of some values
and the implicit disregard of others. These general
considerations are significant with respect to the
assessment of the particular kind of policy that one
devises.

        Second, they identify some general procedural
issues that should be used in developing which values
take priority in adjudicating value conflicts. First,
they suggest that an analysis of the ethics of social
intervention presumes some notion of what values should
apply and how they are to be derived. Minimally, one
can accept the values held by the proponents of the
program. But one could also analyze and evaluate the

values of the group who would be most affected by the
particular intervention. A second issue examines the
weights assigned to the different and frequently competing sets of values held by different groups. This
becomes particularly important in the abortion question.
The survey findings I reported speak to the kinds of
values held by different members of pro and con abortion
groups as well as of the population as a whole. The
other thing that's important to keep in mind with respect to this particular question has to do with the
issue of power. The individuals who have the power to
implement a particular policy may have values that differ considerably from those affected by the policy.
That is, those who will be most affected by a particular
policy may be precisely those who are the least powerful in terms of having their values known, understood,
and respected in terms of developing that policy. The
lack of any significant dialogue between policy makers
and the affected may be one of the most significant
failures of the current policy debate. The third element is the recognition of the value conflicts of the
groups who are engaged in action to achieve a certain
policy. Frequently differences in value priorities set
by different groups will translate into compatible
policy claims and balance in policy become difficult to
achieve. This is especially true when one recalls the
significance of having a variety of single issue groups
associated with a particular cause. Such a coalition
may make the difference between winning or losing a
particular vote on a policy. One needs continuously to
critique the policies proposed by such coalitions of
single issue groups by asking whether they reflect or,
at least, respect the values of those who will be affected by the policy.

5.   Value and Ethical Dilemmas and Problems in the
        Public Policy Debate.

In this section I wish to indicate some of the
problems that I think are critical with respect to the
ethical dimension of the debate over public policy.
These issues clearly relate to and occasionally emerge
from the problems that I have already addressed but
they also go beyond these problems and form a critical
context in which the issues are debated or, more realistically stated, argued.

The first problem is that there are few, if any,
good alternatives to abortion. Adoption clearly is an
alternative to abortion, but choosing adoption requires
that the woman still carry the child to term and deal
with the reality of separation from the newborn, a painful experience even if the woman is highly motivated.
Even in the best of circumstances such a separation will
not easily be made and when there is the suggestion of
coercion or significant familial or other social pressure
to carry the child to term rather than abort, the
separation will be much more problematic.   Even for women who choose to carry a child to term in the expectation of allowing the child to be adopted, there may
be lack of good or even adequate social, physical and
economic support systems to make such a process easier
to accomplish and to insure the health of the mother
and the newborn. Thus as much as a woman may desire to
to have the child adopted, she may not have either the
physical or social support to do so.

Also we need to keep in mind the other alternative to abortion, carrying the child to term and keep-
the child. There are a growing number of women who
choose to keep their babies, especially among the teenage population.[13]   Among the issues here are the ability

and appropriateness of such young mothers' caring for
their child, as well as problems related to adequate
financial and psychological resources to provide an
appropriate setting for the rearing of the child. Often
times teenage mothers need to interrupt their high school
education; they frequently live at home with their parents. These individuals are often already on welfare
or will need such assistance. ˋ In the light of the Reagan
economic philosophy, it appears that reliance on that
particular means of provision will either not be adequate or no longer available.

   Thus even though many individuals see adoption
or the keeping of the child by the mother as preferable to abortion, there are many problems involved in
doing this, especially in light of the unavailability
of social programs to provide a context which would
facilitate these kinds of decisions. Even though a
variety of both counseling programs and economic assistance programs have been made available on a private
basis, these programs are simply not adequate to deal
with all of the needs presented by those individuals
who might wish to carry a child to term and either have
the child adopted or keep their child.

   A second major problem has to do with the perception, if not the reality, of discriminatory treatment
of women who choose abortion.[14] This relates first to
the policy of the federal government which funds both
pre and post natal services under Medicaid. The argument here is that if the government funds these types
of services it should also fund services for abortion.
This position has been argued before the Supreme Court
and the decision was that the government does not discriminate by refusing to provide funds for abortion
under Title 19 of the Social Security Program. Such a

requirement, however, means that such funds cannot come out of the federal budget. It is possible, and in fact many states have continued, to support such abortion programs out of state funds. Nonetheless, Medicaid funded abortions dropped from 295,000 in FY 1977 to about 2,000 in FY 1978.

The other problem that raises the issues of discrimination has to do with the fact that those who will be affected most by cuts in programs will be the poor. Those individuals who are able to afford abortions will continue to be able to afford them, whereas individuals who either cannot afford to have an abortion or who live in states which do not provide funds for abortion may not be able to obtain them. However, one study suggested that the majority of women who wanted an abortion and who would previously have qualified for Medicaid assistance still obtained one. The fiscal, physical, and psychological costs of doing this are not known. Also approximately one-fifth of Medicaid-eligible women were not able to receive abortions because of funding restrictions. Thus the issue is: will a particular group in our society have to bear a disproportionate share of the burden of such funding policies. The consequence of such a policy is that the government's position is not seen as neutral but rather as an aggressive policy designed to decrease the number of abortions. And since it can only do that in cases where it provides the funding, of necessity such restriction have their most significant impact on the poor and the disadvantaged.

There are several subsidiary issues in this problem, among which are determining how abortion fits into the delivery of health care services and the perception that abortion may be a cost effective method

to solve many of the budgetary problems of welfare programs. It is more cost effective to provide abortions
than to provide continuing welfare payments. But such
an observation does not begin to touch or even analyze
the structural arrangements of our society that insure
that a certain number of individuals will always be disenfranchised both politically and economically. We can
also ask what government neutrality with respect to
abortion might mean. Does this mean that the government should not interfere with anyone who wishes to obtain an abortion, or that government should help fund
any health related service a person may want, including
abortion?

A third major issue has to do with the religion-
government relation. One of the major claims of the
pro-abortion groups is that those involved in the antiabortion movement are trying to impose a religious solution to the problem of abortion on those who do not hold
that position and that this violates their religious
freedom. One thing that must be said here has already
wisely been said by Daniel Callahan.[15] That is, there
are religious traditions which approve abortion and, by
that standard, the current policy of liberal abortion
laws in this country is the imposition of a religious
value on another group of people. Also the claims of
foul play do seem to be related only to the abortion
issue. No one is arguing that the religious groups
which are beginning to form coalitions and speak out on
the inherent injustice of the current Reagan economic
program or the immorality of our nuclear deterrence
policy are violating anyone's religious liberty and
that, therefore, they should not engage in these activities.

There are important issues in this debate however. One has to do with how one translates one's religious beliefs or values into language which is appropriate for public debate. That is, is it possible to make insights and values that come from one's religious tradition or experiences accessible to people who do not share those experiences or traditions? The problem here is twofold: being able to make one's self understandable to other individuals and, making the depth of one's convictions accessible and intelligible to individuals who do not stand within that particular tradition. Another issue has to do with one's ecclesiology. How does one see the role of the church with respect to the larger society? Is the church to witness its values to society or is the church to analyze and evaluate, and occasionally reject social values? If one's ecclesiology leads one in the first direction, then it will not be as important to devise a means of translating one's insights so they can be understandable in a broader arena. If one chooses to go the second way, it will be extremely important to develop a language that is widely accessible so that one can easily and helpfully engage in policy debates.

Another issue has to do with the appropriateness of a particular religious group putting itself both ideologically and financially behind a particular cause. Part of the issue here has to do with perceptions about whether a particular religious body has ever done this before and the manner and purpose in which it is perceived to be doing it. I think there is a broad and generally correct perception that the abortion issue is the first time in which the Roman Catholic Church has, to as significant a degree, become involved in both the debate of a public policy issue and has provided rather

large sums of money to help finance different organizations. On the other hand, there seems to be nothing inherently inappropriate about a particular religious body
supporting organizations to advocate a particular point
of view. This is done all the time e.g., the labor
movement, Civil Rights, The Vietnam War, and nuclear
war. The relevant difference in this particular debate
seems to be the fact that it is being done with respect
to abortion and by the Catholic Church. Few comments
seem to be raised about groups and churches that make
financial and ideological contributions to the pro-
abortion half of the debate, or to other political
issues. In fact, I would be willing to argue that the
support of churches, both financially and ideologically,
would be welcomed - if it supported a pro-choice stance
or at least so it seems from reading the list of sponsors
of pro-choice advertisements.

  We need to insist upon some sense of fairness in
discussing churches taking public stands on matters of
significant concern either to them or to the population
at large. The position of a particular church may not
be a popular one, but if it is the position of that
church and there are serious reasons why the church
feels it should engage in fairly direct political action,
then that stance of the church should at least be respected. Often times I think that the real problem is
the perennial one of whose ox is being gored. For
many people, I suspect, as long as the church is sympathetic to their particular position no problems will
be raised. But when the church says something that is
either unpopular or problemmatic, then we tend to think
that the churches should not speak. Such a position is
at best inconsistent and at worst, requires that the
church maintain an inappropriate silence on issues that
the church thinks are of moral significance and political

and social consequence.

The fourth and most significant problem has to do
with how the abortion debate can be conducted in the
public arena. The major issue that I wish to put forward
here, picking up on material developed by MacIntyre and
Hauerwass, is that we, as a culture, have few, if any,
common premises by which we can evaluate and judge competing value claims.

Alistair MacIntyre, in his perceptive article,
"How to Identify Ethical Principles"[16] argues several
theses, one of which is extremely important for the
consideration of ethical issues in the public policy
debate with respect to abortion. His primary claim is
that morality is at war with itself because each moral
agent reaches conclusions by valid forms of inference
but that there is no agreement about the correctness or
appropriateness of the premise with which the argument
begins. MacIntyre then makes an argument that moral
philosophy in general, and I would argue our culture in
particular, has no procedures for weighing rival value
premises. MacIntyre relates this to our cultural and
political background which consists of fragments of a
variety of social philosophies.

There are two major dimensions to this particular
situation. First, we have not inherited the social or
cultural context in which we can both understand and
apply the philosophical theory. Second, we have inherited conflicting theories of ethics or social philosophy.
Thus MacIntyre argues that what we perceive to be the
social-philosophical context out of which our country
developed its political philosophy comes from Aristotle,
Cicero, Locke, and Sidney. Each of these presents conflicting claims with respect to what is good for humans
and, even if one could resolve the epistemological

problems with respect to adjudicating the truth of these different systems, one would still have the practical problem of evaluating the various goods which they claim are in the interests of human beings and the community.

Briefly stated, we have inherited two conflicting world views. First, we have the classical world view which asks the moral question: How might humans together realize the common good? This position assumes that community is natural and normative, there are goods that human beings can rationally identify and agree upon, and that the common pursuit of these will bring both personal and social development. The second claim focuses on the moral question: How may humans prevent each other from interfering with one another as each goes about his or her own concerns? This viewpoint assumes that the state of being autonomous is the appropriate state for human existence, that individuals may not have interests or values in common, and that liberty and the pursuit of interests will maximize individual and social goods.

Our culture and society have attempted to finesse the significant philosophical and ethical problems that come from inheriting a mixed system by developing a liberal society or a pluralistic society. This strategy attempted to take controversial issues out of the political arena and relegate them to the individual conscience. This solution has worked by and large for several generations, but primarily because there was a general acceptance of many of the norms or ideals about human behavior that came out of the classical model. That is, as long as the majority of the citizenry shared a common understanding of what was right and what was wrong and what the limits of individual behavior were, then pluralism could work. Behind pluralism stood a

general understanding of the limits of behavior, even
though this may not have been explicitly articulated or
even socially enforced by the society.

However, we now appear to be in the situation in
which people are attempting to maximize their own freedom and in which the suggestion that some values are
normative appears to be restrictive, coercive, or in an
extreme form, politically repressive. The social sense
seems to be that individuals should pursue their own
interests so long as no one is interfering with anyone
else or no harm is being inflicted on an unconsenting
party. Such a position, generally, stands behind discussions relating to issues of homosexuality, some
aspects of the women's movement, the use of technologies
for fetal screening, heterosexual relationships, and
abortion. Consequently, what we have developing is a
type of moral schizophrenia in which there is some attempt, at least culturally, to hold on to some of the
values and norms that come out of the classical mind
set, while on the other hand having our instinctual
argument arise out of the more modern viewpoint which
argues for the maximization of freedom. Thus, debate
about the merits of a particular action or policy becomes
almost impossible because of the possibly unconscious,
but clearly competing, ethical premises which stand at
the heart of the debate: individual autonomy vs.
community standards.

Thus the ethical political problem is how, in a
culture such as ours in which we have left our common
bonds far behind, can we discuss substantive issues with
profound social consequences. Picture our culture as
a giant circuitry panel. Up to a certain point, the
panel is capable of handling the current load that is
required of it. One can also easily imagine that the
panel can carry a certain amount of overload if one does

a fair degree of creative recircuiting. But the problem
comes when the panel is required to carry a load greater
than that for which it was designed. And at that point
the circuits begin to shut off and the system eventually
burns out. Up until a couple of generations ago, our culture was able to bear the weight of some degree of cultural diversity because the socialization system was
successful in having both the native population and the
immigrants buy into a common value system. But then
over the last couple of decades, beginning probably with
the assassination of Kennedy, the Civil Rights Movement, the Vietnam War, the Feminist Movement, the Gay
Rights Movement, the various urban riots precipitated
both by structural racism and endemic poverty, the rise
and popularity of various religious cults, and now the
abortion question, perhaps the American social system
is reaching the point of circuit overload. We have
been successful to a certain degree in the creative
recircuiting of some of the issues that have been pres-
sing upon us for many years. We can no longer avoid
dealing with these issues. But because we have no commonly accepted framework for analyzing them, we deal
with the issues procedurally by using the judicial system as a means of protecting and promoting individual
rights. Such a maneuver does not evaluate cases on
their merits, but on procedural technicalities precisely
as a way of avoiding the merits of the case. This is
no longer adequate and consequently we are beginning,
I think, to see the signs of a cultural backlash in
which values, which many people may or may not agree
with, are being suggested as appropriate for forming
members of society. We may be in danger of moving
from a culture which has provided for a variability
within certain limits to a culture in which all must

subscribe to the same values and applications of them. The abortion debate may be the first in a series in which revised cultural values are negotiated. If that is the case, the abortion debate may be one of the most significant events of the decade.

Another major issue, and very importantly related to the previous discussion, is how one discusses abortion in the public policy arena from a background of commitment to one's religious position. Such a problem involves two levels at least: one is the problem of translating one's beliefs and values that come from a religious framework into language that can be at least understandable to those who do not share that framework; the second issue relates to one's vision of the role of the church in the large society.

The task of converting one's religious insight into a broader public language is not unique to Christianity. In an early work,[17] John Courtney Murray argued that the fundamental question that the early Christian community had to face was whether insights about Christianity, dependent as they were upon a Judaic framework, could be translated into both a broader cultural and philosophical language. The early community answered this question in the affirmative and the first church councils reflect the translation of Jewish religious concepts into Greek philosophical categories and the history of systematic theology represents the continuation of that translation process. The Catholic church, in particular, has attempted to develop a means of speaking both within and without the church through the philosophical tradition of the natural law. While acknowledging the many theoretical and practical problems in the use of that tradition, nonetheless I think it is important to remember that it

provided a means by which the church could attempt to
conduct a moral and political discourse with those who
did not share the same theological perspectives of the
Catholic community. Using this tradition, Catholic
Christians could speak to the issues of the day in a
language that was accessible to others but whose insights were motivated by a faith tradition.

The problem we have today is: are the categories
of a particular moral tradition sufficient to allow
this kind of discussion to take place? If one assumes
the correctness of the analysis of MacIntyre, then
the natural law tradition is, at best, one viable philosophical tradition among others or, at worst, a carry-
over from a distant age which is no longer viable. Another problem with the natural law tradition is that
while it claimed that it was arguing on rational grounds,
nonetheless the problems, structure, and content of the
arguments were frequently dictated or controlled by a
particular faith stance. Thus although the Catholic
tradition claimed that natural law was a means of
establishing the credibility of a position, frequently
there were situations in which the critical linchpin of
the argument was either the authority of the church or
a faith stance. That awareness makes it difficult to
establish the credibility of one's philosophical argument in the public arena.

This has had at least two significant consequences
for the public arguments against abortion made by many
Catholics. One, the recognition that a philosophical
argument only carries so much weight in the public policy debate has led to the greater use of both faith
statements and ecclesiastical authority to guarantee
one's position. This has reenforced the feeling that
abortion is primarily a religious issue and that the

efforts of the Catholic hierarchy are in many respects
a power play. Too, many Christians, recognizing the
truth of this first consequence, have begun to debate
the abortion issue within the framework of the prochoice
side. This has caused Christians to lose the critical
grounding of their position as well as many of the insights that stem from that ground.[18] Thus their cause
is unnecessarily weakened.

Christians will frequently be at a disadvantage
in the abortion policy debate until they can develop
language and argumentation that respect and incorporate their faith perspective and allows it to be
expressed in such a way that a broader public can
appreciate the position.

Several other issues arise out of differing
perspectives on the role of the church in society,
each of which shapes the policy debate in a unique way.
Several need to be noted: Is the ecclesial tradition
more church oriented or is it more sectarian? Does the
church have a language for and a tradition of speaking
on public policy issues? How has one's church viewed
the complex Constitutional doctrine of the separation
of church and state? What is the history and perception of the history of one's particular ecclesial
tradition with respect to speaking on public policy?
Do the public concerns of the church have more to do
with personal ethics than with social ethics? Do the
publically stated concerns of the church appear to reflect the vested interests of the church or do they
appear to speak to broader social values and concerns?
Finally, while recognizing that there will always be
tension between belief and practice, does the church
provide specific and ample demonstration of how it
promotes both internally and externally the policy that

it articulates for other citizens? That is, does the
church provide a public model for how the policies it
articulates can actually be developed and implemented?

These questions provide a critical examination
of conscience for the churches to engage in as they
both argue their positions on abortion and recommend a
public policy consistens with those positions. This
examination will not guarantee that a church develop a
correct policy or that it develop the best policy.
What the examination may help ensure is that Christians
be more civil in their conducting of the debate and more
coherent and consistent in how they reconcile their
beliefs with the realities of the process for establishing public policy. The churches have an important role
in establishing policy and should be insistent upon
exercising this role even in the face of opposition
from both within and from without.

Thus, it is not enough for the church to be a
kind of "contrast model", as Hauerwass suggests or to
be an agent of "critical negativity" as Schillebeeckx
calls for, or even a political lobby as the National
Rifle Association. Without claiming that the church
has final word on a particular social demonstration
of a faith statement, it is nonetheless critical and
of ultimate significance that the church live out what
it professes. If the church cannot from within provide
convincing examples and models of the behavior it argues
as appropriate public policy, then that policy will
be perceived as bankrupt, impossible to actualize, or
an example of social control in a most pejorative sense.
In the Catholic Christian tradition, there has always
been a strong sense of the need to look to the witness
of belief in the community as a source of belief. It
is here where we must look for the models on the basis

of which policy can be suggested for the broader community. By modeling a particular policy and demonstrating its possibilities and viability, the church has
the possibility of being truly for others a servant to
others, and in this way influencing policy in a way that
no interest group possibly could.

6.   Conclusions.

        To speak in these idealistic terms of the church
is not, I hope, to be ignorant of the costs of the
church's modeling a particular behavior or of the
church's problems in defining and actualizing a particular policy. The costs of attempting to devise even
a moderate policy on abortion have been particularly
clearly spelled out in a recent article by Peter
Steinfels.[19] Steinfels suggests that there are two
steps that this group should take, each of which involves a break with one or the other sides of the
current debate. The first step argues that psychological, social, and even religious incentives that
disapprove of abortion will be insufficient to restrict
effectively severe attacks on the value of fetal life.
This argument suggests that some legislative restrictions are necessary to protect the value of life and
that, some women, though Steinfels argues not all,
would have to carry a pregnancy to term. Such a
position will be difficult for Catholic feminists and
liberals - as well as many others. This option gives
a high value to fetal life and recognizes that some
social supports in the form of restrictive legislation
are necessary to protect that life.

        The second step requires liberal Catholics to
break with the pro-life movement by arguing that the
ethical status of the fetus is a difficult moral problem, especially in the very early stages of the develop-

ment of the embryo. While one can argue that even from
the earliest moments of conception the conceptus is a
member of the human species and is alive, it is difficult to prove in a convincing way that at that time the
developing embryo has all of the rights to the preservation and protection of life as a newborn, as a child,
or as an adult. The recognition of the moral ambiguity
surrounding the status of the embryo would allow room
to maneuver when developing a policy on abortion. But
it would require a significant degree of ethical compromise for some, perhaps many, members of different
churches.

     What is important about Stenfels' argument is not
whether or not his reading of policy on abortion is
correct, but the fact that he has thought through the
significant compromises that will need to be made in
terms of establishing some kind of policy that has a
chance of being viable, one that permits abortion up
to 8 weeks of the pregnancy. And one condition of
viability for that particular policy is that two specific populations, pregnant women and fetuses, will have
to suffer as a consequence. Members of different groups
will experience moral compromise but clearly not as
much as pregnant women and fetuses. Compromise is seldom easy, and it will be far less easy when one recognizes that a policy may require that some women carry
an unwanted pregnancy to term and that some fetuses
will be aborted.

     In addition to compromise, I think that it is
also important for the churches to recognize that in
many ways the tone and style of the debate over abortion is being set by extremes on both ends of the
spectrum. If one refers to some of the data about the
perceptions on abortion in both the National Rights to
Life Committee and the National Abortion Rights Action

League that I have mentioned, it may be the case that
there is room for some maneuvering with respect to public policy, as long as neither of these two groups gets
its way. That is a rather harsh statement, but I think
it is important to recognize that even within the NRLC
there are members who will allow abortion under some
circumstances and in NARAL there are individuals who
do not think that all reasons for abortion are morally
significant. What we need to begin paying attention to
is not the rhetoric of the groups or the claims to
purity of doctrine, but what the real beliefs of individuals in these organizations are, in addition to
listening to what the real beliefs of members of different churches are. ˉMy sense is that as long as policy is defined by either extreme or some other single
interest group, no progress can be made because the
policy defined by these groups will be so extreme that
a viable coalition based on actual beliefs and practice
cannot support it, nor can legislation be developed
that recognizes both diversity of opinion and broad
areas of consensus.

    In addition to compromise and a policy based on
the realistic beliefs of the population, whether those
be political or religious, it is also important for
the society, if it truly believes in the value of life
and fetal life in particular, to begin providing
structures which make it possible for individuals to
act on this belief. Such an orientation would require
on the one hand a high degree of fairness and coherence
among a variety of policies and would in effect, suggest that funding be provided for both abortions and
pre and post natal care. Minimal fairness requires, I
think, that provision be made for people to act out
their particular choices. There is a genuine problem

here and a real danger. Clearly abortion is more cost
effective than the provision of a variety of social services. However, I still find it reprehensible to think
that abortion is the solution to a variety of social
problems that have to do with the health care of pregnant women, the ability of families to provide adequate
food, shelter and education for their children, as well
as a minimal standard of a quality of life. I also need
to recognize that however optimally our social structures
may be arranged, there always will be, I think, the
need for abortion. My hope is that a moderately restrictive policy on abortion together with the availability of contraceptives and reasonable social policies to support women and couples who wish to have children might permit a genuine moral debate to occur about
having an abortion in a particular situation.

Public policy on abortion must be seen as: a
part of a larger policy having to do with the status
of individual choice within a pluralistic community; a
respect for differing and often contradictory value
systems professed by members of the larger society, both
as private individuals and as members of various voluntary associations including the churches; a recognition
that there is a large enough middle ground between the
extremes upon which to make a reasonable appeal for a
moderate policy on abortion; a respect for fetal life,
but which must be rooted in the recognition that there
are moral problems in establishing an inviolable right
to life for the fetus; and finally, as respecting the
different positions of the churches, but with the
recognition that their public policy recommendations be
tested against their beliefs and actions.

There can be a responsible public policy debate
on abortion, but only if we are willing to bear the burden of compromise and the responsibility of realizing
that wherever a line is drawn, that line will entail
hardship and that we as a community must be willing to
provide as best we can for those individuals who must
bear the burden of a particular public policy.[20]

FOOTNOTES

1. Christopher Tietze, Induced Abortion: A World Review, 1981. N.Y.: The Population Council. p. 1.

2. Ibid., p. 5.

3. Ibid., pp. 34-35.

4. James C. Mohr, Abortion In America. N.Y.: Oxford University Press, 1978. pp. 20-45.

5. Ibid., pp. 250-255.

6. Raymond Tatalovich and Byron W. Daynes, "The Trauma of Abortion Politics." Commonweal 107 (20 Nov. 1981), pp. 644-649.

7. Donald Granberg and Beth Wellman Granberg. "Abortion Attitudes, 1965-1980: Trends and Determinants." Family Planning Perspectives. 12 (Sept./Oct., 1980), pp. 251-252.

8. Ibid., p. 252.

9. Ibid., pp. 253-258.

10. Donald Granberg, "The Abortion Activists." Family Planning Perspectives. (13 July/August, 1981) pp.157-163.

11. James Kelly, "Beyond the Stereotypes." Commonweal 107 (20 Nov. 81), pp. 654-659.

12. Herbert C. Kelmun and Donald P. Warwick, "The Ethics of Social Intervention: Goals, Means, and Consequences." In Policy Studies Review Annual, Bertram H. Raven, Ed. Beverly Hills: Sge Publications, 1980. pp. 44-46.

13. Perihan A. Rosenthal, "Adolescence and Pregnancy", Department of Psychiatry, University of Massachu-setts Medical Center. Unpublished manuscript. Richard P. Perkins and others, "Intensive Care in Adolescent Pregnancy." Obstetrics and Gynecology 52 (August, 1978), pp. 179-188.

14. The perception certainly approaches reality when one hears Senator Hyde, who sponsored legislation to restrict abortions paid for by Medicaid to those which threatened the life of the woman, say: "I certainly would like to prevent, if I could legally, anybody having an abortion, a rich woman, a middle-class woman or a poor woman. Unfortunately, the only vehicle available is the HEW Medicaid bill. A life is a life." The Congressional Record 17 June, 1977. p. H 6083. Quoted from Family Planning Perspectives 12 (May/June, 1980) p. 121.

15. Daniel Callahan, "Abortion: Some Ethical Issues." In Bioethics, Ed. T. A. Shannon. N.Y.: Paulist Press. 1981 (Revised Edition). p. 16.

16. Alasdair MacIntyre, "How to Identify Ethical Principles." The Belmont Report, Appendix, Volume I. DHEW Publication No. (OS) 78-0013. 10-1-41.

17. John Courtney Murray. The Problem of God. New Haven: Yale University Press. 1964 pp. 31ff.

18. Stanley Hawerwass, A Community of Character. Notre Dame: The University of Notre Dame Press. 1981. p. 213.

19. Peter Steinfels, "The Search for an Alternative." Commonweal 107 (20 Nov., 1981) pp. 660-664

20. Much of the material in this essay was originally published in Abortion and the Status of the Fetus, W. Bondeson et al. Eds., D. Reidel Publishing Co., 1983, and is reprinted with their permission.

ETHICAL IMPLICATIONS
OF DEVELOPMENTS IN GENETICS

I.   Introduction

   A. Purpose

   The overall purpose of this chapter is to describe
contemporary developments in genetics that have raised
a variety of ethical problems. To do this, I will describe several of these developments, raise some of the
thematic ethical issues to which they point, and describe
some of the responses that have been made to them.
Therefore, I wish to look at two broad problem areas
related to the application of specific knowledge and
to the implications of gaining such knowledge in the
field of genetics. My intent in discussing the ethical
dimension of these problems is to provide an overview
of the debates that are occurring with respect to these
problem areas. Thus, I am more interested in presenting the contours of the debate rather than argue specific points, although that will also occur. I think it
is also important to note that several of the specific
problems I discuss are linked together. I want to
separate several of these primarily for purposes of
discussion and analysis.

   B. Definitions

   Genetics is the division of the life sciences that
focuses exclusively on the genes or the units that determine one's inheritance. Occasionally in bio-ethical
discussions, genetics is used as a shorthand way of
referring to many of the disciplines and developments
within the life sciences. Although I will occasionally
use the word in this broad sense, I will primarily

be using it in the technical sense of the study of the genes and the application of that knowledge in a variety of settings. The genes are the basic blueprint or plan for heredity, the program which helps specify how an organism will develop. The genes are made up of segments of DNA, deoxyribonucleic acid, in which four chemical subunits are united in a variety of ways. These four chemicals, abbreviated as A, G, C, T, are the alphabet which carries to the cell the instructions for making proteins. Within recent years, geneticists have learned more and more about the composition of this alphabet, the processes by which the message is originally written and communicated, and the ways in which the messages can be read. Such growing understanding of the genetic code has occasioned many discussions of the problems of both application and implication that find their way into this chapter.

The term genetic engineering has a similar narrow and broad meaning. Strictly speaking, it refers to specific technical interventions into the structure of a gene for a variety of purposes including, but not limited to, removing a deleterious gene, changing the genetic structure of a particular organism, or enhancing a particular genetic capacity. Genetic engineering is a specific intervention into the actual genetic structure itself. In a broader sense, and in the sense most often used, genetic engineering refers to the possibility of designing not only our descendants, but also of manipulating the entire ecosystem in specific directions. More specifically, though, genetic engineering in the broad sense refers to technologies such as in vitro fertilization, cloning, recombinant DNA research, and a variety of other applications of the knowledge of genetics that has a social or policy dimension.

C.   Method

To accomplish the end of presenting several developments in genetics and genetic engineering that have
ethical implications, I am going to describe two general
problematic issues in genetics - application and implication, present the elements in the ethical debate,
and provide both a framework for discussion and a bibliographical essay.

II.   Problems of Application

A.   The Technologies

Recombinant DNA research is basically a technique
by which a segment of DNA can be removed from its original strand and joined to another segment of DNA from
a different organism, thus forming the recombinant molecule. The new DNA that is placed into the host begins
to replicate itself there. Thus, for example, a molecule
can be made to produce insulin, a new species or organism
could be devised or a new pathogenetic agent could be
made for use in insect control or biological-chemical
warfare.

Amniocentesis is a technique in which fetal cells
are withdrawn from the amniotic fluid in the uterus by
means of a needle inserted through the pregnant woman's
abdomen. These fetal cells are then cultured,
and the chromosomes are screened to determine whether
or not the developing embryo has a genetic anomaly.
Several hundred genetic diseases can be diagnosed in
utero and the sex of the fetus can be determined.
This technique is almost risk-free for both the mother
and the fetus and, given reasonable standards of quality
control in the laboratory, is a highly reliable diagnostic technique.

In vitro fertilization and embryo transplant, or external human fertilization, received a great deal of attention in 1978 when the first baby conceived, transplanted and delivered by such a process was born in England. This technology involves removal of an egg from the ovary, external fertilization and then implantation into a prepared uterus. While a fairly straightforward procedure, the success of this technique involves the interlocking of a variety of developments in an understanding of the hormonal processes that control the female reproductive cycle, the development of a proper culture in which to have the fertilization occur as well as the development of safe and reliable techniques for the removal of the egg and the transfer of the blastocyte.

B.   Ethical Issues

1.   Science and Society.   One of the critical issues in this area is that of how science is perceived. two important viewpoints are provided by contemporary comentators.   Pope John Paul II, in his first encyclical letter "Redemptor hominis",[1] suggested that humans are becoming afraid of what they produce because of the perception that these products could radically turn against themselves.   He emphasizes the growing fear that our products can become the means and instruments for self-destruction.   Pope John Paul then asks why it is that this power has turned against humans and produced a state of disquiet, of fear and menace. Part of the answer that he suggests comes from a shift in persons perceiving themselves not as masters or guardians of the world but as its exploiters and destroyers.   Coupled with this is the issue of determining whether or not those things which are produced make life more human and, therefore, more worthy of persons.

Another perspective is presented by Daniel
Callahan[2] who reports that current developments in
genetic engineering, broadly speaking, suggest that both
the scientific community and the general public are more
prepared than ever to go ahead with new developments.
Callahan indicates that there has been a typical reaction of wonder and excitement in both the scientific
and public media whenever a major breakthough has been
discovered. He concludes that society continues to be
attracted to scientific progress and technological applications of new insights into the processes of nature.
Callahan suggests that such a posture continues because
no generally persuasive argument against continued research
and development in genetics has been developed. By this
he means that there has been no argument that goes beyond logic to an emotional attractiveness that could
impel people to act or not act. That is, none of the
arguments against genetic engineering have been able to
touch any of our cultural, ethical or religious values
in a way that is relevant to a critical evaluation of
genetic engineering. Because of this, business has
continued fairly much as usual and appears likely to do
so for the foreseeable future.

This model is changing, primarily because of
discoveries in genetics as well as the application of
a variety of other scientific principles, especially that
of nuclear power. The new perception is that not only
can we know the truths of nature but we can also change
nature. The discovery of the structure of DNA by Watson
and Crick in the early 1950's set in motion a chain of
events that has led to the technique of recombinant DNA.
It is now possible, as mentioned previously, to recons-
truct various molecules and to make them perform in new
ways. It is equally possible to build a new species

out of previously existing species and in this way directly intervene in the evolutionary process. In addition
to being able to state the basic scientific laws that
regulate the workings of nature, it is also possible to
intervene into the very heart of the genetic code to
change the information and produce a new product.

Such powers, of course, raise a variety of
issues related to social implications of such a shift in
model. One of the major areas in impact will be on the
self-understanding of the scientist. Although the cari-
cature of the scientist sitting in the research laboratory, unencumbered by any of the cares of the workaday
world is manifestly inaccurate, nonetheless many scientists direct their primary efforts to basic research
with little worry of potential applications or of long-
term implications of what they are doing. It was assumed that they were apolitical and primarily providing
a service which society would determine how to use.

In the light of the new possibilities within
science, however, such a posture may no longer be adequate. At least, a scientist must re-examine what is
the nature of the profession of science and what its
relation to society might be. Callahan has suggested
four general propositions which are helpful in such an
initial re-evaluation.

> 1.   Individuals and groups are ordinarily
> responsible for only the consequences of those
> actions if, through negligence, they fail to
> take into account such consequences.

2.   Individuals and groups cannot be held responsible for those actions the consequences of which are totally unknown. However, if they voluntarily undertake such acts, they may be held responsible for the consequences unless there were serious reasons for undertaking action in the first place. One cannot, without serious reason, just "play around" in the unknown while simultaneously disclaiming responsibility for the results.

3.   When others may be affected by our actions, they ordinarily have a right to demand that their wishes and values be respected. This is particularly the case when those actions may result in harm to them.

4.   Individual scientists and scientific groups are subject to the same norms of ethical responsibility as those of all other individuals in groups in society. They have neither more responsibility for their actions nor less; there is no special ethic of responsibility applying to scientists that does not apply to others.[4]

Callahan then supplements these general propositions with two principles that he derives from the basis of our past experience. The first of these is what he calls the historical principle. This principle suggests that we know, in ways that earlier generations did not, that the search for knowledge can bring about harmful consequences and that it is possible to trace back the causal sequence. Because we know this is possible from past experience, Callahan argues that we should evaluate more carefully research that can set in motion causal chains, of which some outcomes might conceivably be

harmful. This historical principle is supplemented with
the imagination principle which suggests that a scientist
might well assume that since unintended harmful consequences have happened with other forms of research, he or
she might assume that the same thing could happen with
this particular project. Therefore, it is incumbent on
the scientist to try to imagine ahead or to envision
possibilities that may arise in the outcomes of the
particular project so that they can be evaluated personally and socially. Such a framework, while not
totally fail-safe, provides at least a context in which
critical evaluation can occur before a project is
started or when it appears that there may be harmful outcomes of a particular application of knowledge from a
project.

The past debate over the safety of recombinant
DNA research and the growing debate over the safety of
nuclear power has brought forth a new model of a
scientist: the scientist as advocate. In these debates,
we see different scientists hurling technical as well
as personal accusations against one another. The problem
that is revealed is the possibility that experts in a
field can and do disagree on both the facts and the interpretation of those facts. The disagreement, however,
allowed scientists to be perceived by the public and
their peers as advocates for a particular position or
cause. Many scientists realized that they were in a
new role and were often uncomfortable with it; they also
realized that many of the issues that they were discussing were socially important enough to justify such a
shift in role. Of course, the model of the scientist
as advocate presents an interesting problem about the
relationship between facts and values. Oftentimes the
facts may be reasonably clear and apparent, but the

framework for the evaluation of these facts may be quite different between scientists for a variety of personal and social reasons. For example, one scientist may be willing to accept different risks than another and this will color how he or she evaluates a particular problem. Thus, it is important for the scientist, when he or she assumes the role of advocate, to recognize as clearly as possible the personal, scientific, social and cultural sources of his or her viewpoint so that the advocacy can be on as reasonable a basis as possible.

2.   Nature and Ethics. The second major area of discussion that is raised by some developments in genetics is the relationship between nature and ethics. One of the traditional viewpoints in this discussion is to see nature as a type of limit. I suggest the traditional natural law philosophy as an example of this perspective. In this tradition, one uses the order of nature as the basis upon which one elucidates moral principles. This is justified because the order of nature reflects the plan of God for nature which can be discovered and understood by human reason. Because this order of nature is normative, one can legitimately argue that nature in this perspective is a conservative or limiting principle. That is, it sets up limits or bounds beyond which one may not go. As an example we can refer to the traditional argument against the use of artificial contraceptives which, in simplified form, states that they separate what nature united - sexual intercourse and procreation. Such a unity, it is argued, is inherent in the order of nature which reflects divine reason and, therefore, this structure limits what can be done in this area. Such a moral tradition tends to be conservative and would approach some interventions into nature with caution, if not suspicion.

A second perspective envisions nature as a model. This orientation, similar to the natural law perspective mentioned above, argues that we can replicate some occurences in nature. While this model may not allow any more interventions into nature than the previously discussed model would, it would certainly expand the kinds of things one could do on the basis of nature. In this framework, it might be legitimate to replicate certain instances of premoral evils that occur in nature as long as one has a proportionate reason for so doing. For example, it is the case that a fairly high number of zygotes are lost during the first several weeks of the process of conception and implantation and initial development. A number of these zygotes seem to be naturally aborted because of structural anomalies, hormonal imbalances within the uterus, or a variety of other problems connected with the necessity of many different systems coming together at precisely the right moment. Would it be legimate, therefore, to replicate this instance of embryo loss in a laboratory during the course of efforts to fertilize human ova in vitro? A great number of research protocols could be justified in terms of the benefits both to future embryos and fetuses as well as the possibility of bringing benefits to those women who are unable to conceive in any other way. In this framework one would be replicating a natural phenomenon in the laboratory and justifying the pre-moral evil of embryonic loss on the basis of the benefits to be achieved by the research or the pregnancy, just as the high number of embryonic loss is justified in nature by the goods of family and children.

Such an argument is put forward by Richard McCormick who limits its application to efforts to achieve a pregnancy. He says: "It is not a violation of the right to life of the zygote if it is spontaneously lost in normal sexual relations. Why is it any more so when this loss occurs as the result of an attempt to achieve pregnancy artificially?"[5] Karl Rahner, basing his orientation of the doubtfulness of the personhood of the fertilized ovum, suggests that zygotes could be used as subjects of experimentation. "But it would be conceivable that, given a serious positive doubt about the human quality of the experimental material, the reasons in favor of experimenting might carry more weight, considered rationally, than the uncertain rights of a human being whose very existence is in doubt."[6]

This orientation is countered by Leon Kass. But although he takes a very strong stand against the use of embryos for research, he seems to allow the possibility of their use in research that leads to a pregnancy.

> Parenthetically, we should note that the natural occurence of embryo and fetal loss and wastage does not necessarily or automatically justify all deliberate, humanly caused destruction of fetal life. For example, the natural loss of embryos in early pregnancy cannot in itself be a warrant for deliberately aborting them or for invasively experimenting on them in vitro any more than stillbirths could be a justification for newborn infanticide. There are many things that happen naturally that we ought not to do deliberately. It is curious how the same people who deny the relevance of nature as a guide for re-evaluating

human interventions into human generation,
and who deny that the term "unnatural"
carries any ethical weight, will themselves appeal to "nature's way" when it
suits their purposes. Still, in this
present matter, the closeness to natural
procreation - the goal is the same, the
embryonic loss is unavoidable and not
desired, and the amount of loss is
similar - leads me to believe that we
do no more intentional or unjustified
harm in the one case than in the other,
and practice no disrespect.[7]

The third model of nature defines nature as
evolving. The first two models of nature that I presented
basically assume that nature is reasonably static and
that the order that is present will remain. This model
of nature sees nature as continually evolving. This
does not necessarily imply that there is no stability
to nature or no laws of nature that can be known. It
does suggest, however, that such laws and structures may
not be as normative as the other models would suggest
and that a much greater degree of intervention may be
possible. This view, for example, would see change and/
or development as normative rather than exceptional.
The working assumption of this model is that things
change, and that they change with respect to broader
developments within the ecosystem as a whole.

Within this model the concept of history takes
on an importance lacking in the other two models.
History here is seen as linear or teleological, rather
than cyclic or episodic. History has a future, and
that future carries history forward. In Christianity,
this orientation contains a dichotomy: the ultimate

future transcends persons and their efforts at self
creation but, through their interventions in history and
nature, persons open themselves to this future and help
to achieve it. As Rahner says: "This human self-creation
will develop the concrete form of human openness which
leads to the absolute future that comes from God. But
it is never capable by itself of bringing about this
absolute future. Christianity, precisely because it is
the religion of the absolute future must simultaneously
send man out to his duties in the world."[8]

It is clear that future developments are not entirely knowable or predictable. Yet, on the other hand,
we know that we are evolving and that we have an increasing capacity to determine various directions of
evolution, including human evolution. Thus, developments in genetics, as well as in psychology, psychiatry
and many of the behavioral sciences have made it possible to intervene in the development of human beings,
and possibly into human nature, in a way never before
thought possible. The previous two models suggested
that nature may serve either as a limit or as a mirror
of the kinds of interventions that might be ethically
possible. Nature will not necessarily have such limiting capabilities in an evolutionary model because the
past will not necessarily possess qualities necessary
to insure survival in the future. The past is no longer
normative and the future assumes a greater role in
defining efforts at self-creation. Such a possibility
leaves us caught between the attempt to determine how
much of our own self-perception and understanding of
our nature is tied to our biology and place within the
ecosystem and history, and the perception that we
possess the powers to change the course of the direction
of evolution in accordance with our desires and

preferences. In this model, a variety of interventions becomes possible and will be justified in terms of survival value, adaptability and promotion of a model of human nature that is seen as desirable.

3.   Problems of Knowledge. A third major problem area is that associated with problems of knowledge. We have all known the pains and anguish that come from knowing too little, especially about how to cure a particular disease that is killing an individual. Lack of knowledge often makes us helpless to solve a particular problem or to know how to develop a variety of strategies to provide for different contingencies. Limited knowledge has also made individuals hold on much too securely to that which is known for fear that if that is questioned the foundations will be shaken and the universe will collapse. Limited knowledge can lead to a repression of knowledge and we all know the terror that comes when the pursuit of knowledge is repressed.

In our day we have the problem of seemingly too much knowledge. The information explosion has caused facts, as well as the journals and books that report these facts, to proliferate at a rate which makes it impossible for a responsible professional to keep track of new developments, even within a very narrowly defined area of knowledge. Another problem associated with this information explosion relates to the qualitative dimension of that information. We are beginning to ask, and in many ways are being forced to ask, questions to which we really have neither a good answer nor a sense of how to go about answering the question. Our traditional sources of values are being strained to their limits by our technical capacities that follow from our gains in knowledge. A variety of disciplines including genetics, psychology, psychiatry, philosophy and theology have all coalesced to raise questions about the meaning of the human. Until fairly recently most of us were reasonably satisfied that we had a workable sense of who we were and what we were about. New discoveries and insights into the full range of possible meanings of the human have given us a new burden in that we are no longer quite sure of who we are or what we are to be about. The culture in which we live certainly reinforces this questioning but perversely casts us further adrift because it provides neither a common basis nor a set of values which can help provide a firm foundation on which to begin to construct a new answer to the question of what is a human being.

In addition to these problems relating to knowledge, a third major issue is beginning to arise: discussions of the possibility of limiting or restricting research. Freedom of speech and freedom of thought are, of course, two of the most cherished values of our American culture and serve as significant ethical values in many theories of ethics. Any suggestion that knowledge be restrained faces a most difficult challenge. In fact, the presumption is that any restriction on knowledge or thought is almost inherently evil. Yet if one keeps in mind the shift in the model of nature from one of discovering the truth to that of changing nature, the argument may change somewhat. The knowledge that is in question here is knowledge of application or knowledge of implication.

Few people argue that scientists should be restrained in thinking through a particular problem or speculating on a new theory. The traditional argument for this position is well stated by Key Dismukes: "A major factor in advancing scientific understanding and correcting error is the opportunity of critics to

challenge prevailing views and, if they can adduce
convincing evidence, to modify an existing consensus.
This aspect of science is more than a convenient and
useful tradition. It is essential to the operation of
science as freedom of speech is to the maintenance of
democracy."[9]

The critical problem arises, however, when such
knowledge is applied or is translated into action. Here
the lines are not so cleanly drawn, although there is
the tradition in American law that, for example, religious freedom is limited to a freedom to believe whatever
one wants, but not a similar freedom to act upon those
beliefs. Some restrictions on actions are already in
place, such as regulations concerning the participation
of human subjects in biomedical and behavioral research
and the regulations concerning the recombinant DNA
technology.

One background issue in this discussion is the
fact that progress has become an important value within
our society. In many ways the knowledge explosion is
a direct result of our valuing progress. The unconscious
or uncritical assumption is that progress is in and of
itself valuable and therefore must be pursued. To
achieve this goal, research and development is necessary and has a high priority. But it is legimate at
least to question the value of progress and its role
in our society, even though General Electric may continue to argue that it is our most important product.
If progress is not morally necessary and perhaps
optional, then it may be the case that a lot of what
we perceive to be necessary may be interesting but
superfluous. This is not a direct argument against
the concept and reality of progress itself; it is a
suggestion that mindless progress with its exponential

generation of data may be inappropriate at this time.
This is especially so in the light of diminishing resources,
especially money and energy. At a time when the total
budget to be spent on scientific research and development
is diminishing, it may be appropriate to target certain
areas of research as having priority because of their
social necessity and value. In this light, limitations on
research and knowledge could come about, not because of
inherent distrust of the knowledge to be gained or problems
with its application, but rather because of the acceptance
of a new system of social values and priorities. Greater
care in the selection of research projects to fund would
of necessity limit knowledge both quantitatively and
qualitatively.

Yet, as Daniel Callahan indicates, our society at
present values both basic scientific research and applied
scientific research.[10] Because of this cultural value,
he argues that the burden of proof must lie with those
who are opposed to research. He makes two exceptions to
this basic rule. The first would arise in a case where
serious potential harm to the general public can be hypothesized with a degree or probability greater than 0.
When that is the case those who wish to pursue the research
must submit the issue to the public discussion and judgment. A second exception arises when there is a high probability that harm would result from the basic research
which would be of a magnitude such as to pose serious
threats to human welfare. In that instance, Callahan
argues that the research should not go forward at all,
even if it would be supported by the public. Such an
orientation, building as it does on the current cultural
status quo, is persuasive in its argument that the burden
of proof rests with those who are opposed to research.
Yet it does allow for the possibility of restricting research when there is a probability of harm and of pro-

hibiting research when there would be serious harm to human welfare. Although not foolproof and containing several ambiguities, such a position allows the discussion of this critical issue within our contemporary social framework.

In a recent article, David Smith suggests several reasons for restricting freedom of inquiry.[11] The first of these argues that knowledge may be immoral in its use and, therefore, may be restricted. This position would argue that the right to know must be less than absolute because some knowledge can end up doing more harm than good. While recognizing the problems and limitations with this orientation, Smith thinks that it is important to think through what consequences the use of knowledge will have. He also suggests that knowledge that is either obtained or disseminated in an immoral way should be restricted. Here he argues that knowledge obtained at the expense of violating a person's integrity or privacy is immoral and such attempts to gain knowledge by these means should be restricted. He also argues here that knowledge which is disseminated in a way that is destructive of just cultural institutions or practices is immoral and should be restrained because it threatens the very fabric and basis of our life together. Finally, Smith suggests that knowledge which can be destructive of us as persons should be restricted. Some knowledge could shatter a person's world view, and Smith argues that perhaps that knowledge should not be communicated to that person. He also suggests that premature communication of scientific theories could be immoral because they are untimely and therefore may also be harmful to a person's self understanding. The basis of Smith's argument is his perception that knowledge is social and must be evaluated in a social context, not in exclusively individualistic framework. He also argues that a scholar or scientist has some responsibility for the repercussions of his or her

speaking the truth and that, therefore, they should evaluate what they are saying, when they are saying it, and
why they are saying it before they actually do say it.
Thus, Smith concludes by arguing for a tradition of self-
disciplined hesitation rather than censorship or repression.

III.   Problems of Implication

　　A.　The Technologies

　　One of the major spin-offs of our understanding
of genetics has been the development of programs of
genetic screening in which carriers of a variety of
genetic diseases can be identified and information
given to them so they can make a more informed reproductive decision. Such screening programs involve an
identification of a target population and an examination
of the chromosomes of the individuals in the population to determine whether or not they contain deleterious
genes. Then the information is given to the individual,
and further genetic counseling can be obtained if desired.

　　Another area that is of growing importance is
genetic engineering in which a variety of therapies will
be initiated by replacing or removing deleterious genes
from an individual so that a disease will not occur or
will be corrected. The technology of recombinant DNA
also makes it possible to envision the development of
new species. Future developments offer the possibility
of intervening directly into an individual's genetic
structure for reasons of therapy or the achievement of
personal or social desires.

　　Another area of implication in genetics is really
not a technology but an initial formulation of an academic discipline: sociobiology. This is the systematic
study of the biological basis of all forms of social
behavior in all kinds of organisms including humans.
This new discipline is important because of the far-
reaching questions it raises about the sources of

various kinds of human behavior, especially altruism and
freedom. The implications of such questioning of these
values forms of human behavior raises significant questions that need to be addressed at least in a preliminary
fashion in a session such as this.

    B.   Ethical Issues

    1.   Definitions of Health. One of the critical,
thematic issues that is raised by both genetic screening
programs and by genetic engineering is the question of what
is health and what is disease. Such a discussion is extremely relevant because definitions of health and disease provide the baseline for a medical and ethical argument to
determine whether or not intervention is appropriate. One
can argue, for example, that definitions of health and
disease should be mainly physiological.[12] That is, one
should view health as functional normality which looks to
function according to design, to conformity and goals pursued by the organism, as well as the working out of the
design of the organism. This orientation suggests that
each structure or organ of the body has a particular range
of activities and that if there is a deviation from that
range, there is the possibility of a disease. If that disease becomes disabling, then it becomes an illness. This
makes the task of diagnosis fairly simple.

    This perspective is being incorporated into an ethi-
cal argument by Paul Ramsey who proposed that the first
level of analysis should be what he calls a medical indications policy.[13] Here Ramsey argues that a decision to
treat or not to treat should be made primarily on the basis
of physiological criteria. That is, in determining whether
or not there is an obligation to treat or not to treat, the
baseline is the determination of whether this treatment wil
benefit the patient or not. Such an ethical baseline
rests on a physiological definition of health and

disease, as well as the presumption that such determination can be made in a primarily value-free context.

A second orientation argues that definitions of health and disease, in addition to a psychological dimension, also contain a cultural or social component. This is especially true in the areas of psychology and psychiatry, although it is also relevant to the evaluation of genetic diseases. For example, it is relatively easy to diagnose a broken arm and have little, if any, disagreement about the problem; the same is true about a variety of other illnesses. On the other hand, when one is attempting to determine whether one is deviant, crazy or normal, the task is quite difficult and is open to a variety of interpretations based on both one's psychiatric theory as well as one's cultural and social values. While I accept and would argue that there certainly is such a reality as mental illness, I think it is imperative at the same time to recognize that there is a high component of both ideological biases and cultural values that influence how we perceive individuals whose behavior is seemingly outside the range of what is either accepted as normal or socially approved.

Such issues can affect an individual with a genetic disease in a variety of ways. It is clear that the phenomenon of Down's syndrome is heritable and that individuals who have the syndrome suffer among other things a diminished capacity for abstract reasoning. There are clear physiological criteria by which one can diagnose the disease, and there are also psychological markers by which one can determine the degree of retardation. Yet that is not the end of the story, for intelligence is highly valued within our society and puts the diagnosis of this syndrome into a different category.

One who has this particular genetic disease is seen as a different kind of individual. He or she is one who does not merely have a disease; this individual is also socially impaired and disvalued.

Others suggest that knowledge of an individual's genetic constitution may significantly alter how that individual is raised. For example, several individuals possess the XYY syndrome, which physiologically is simply the presence of an extra Y chromosome. One of the early suggestions in the literature about the social effects of this syndrome was that it was a possible predictor of aggressive or antisocial behavior. If parents were to learn that their child was affected with this syndrome and that there was the possibility of this syndrome causing anti-social behavior, could this not significantly alter how the parents raise the boy? Should the parents perceive this child as healthy or ill, diseased or well? Regardless of how one answers these questions, we have here an example of a genetic anomaly that has a clear physiological criterion but an unclear social outcome with respect to its effects on the child. The way in which this boy will be raised may be in large part dependent upon whether one uses primarily physiological or primarily cultural norms to evaluate his state of health.

Another area of impact is the often unclear distinc-tion between one who is a carrier of a disease and one who is afflicted with the disease. Being a carrier of a disease does not imply that one has the symptoms of the disease or is afflicted by the disease in any way. Genetic screening programs discover both those individuals who are carriers of a disease as well as those who are afflicted with it. If the distinction between such individuals is misunder-stood or confused and communicated in this fashion to others such as insurance companies, individuals who are only carriers of a disease could be prevented from receiving insurance policies or other

health care benefits because it would be assumed that
they were unhealthy. Not only are such individuals
unjustly deprived of health care benefits, but they
are unfairly labeled, and this provides a possible
basis for discriminatory treatment.

2. Perception of Self and One's Descendants.
A second problem involved the perception of one's self
and one's descendants. The traditional ethical model
in which personal responsibility was exercised in relation to the earth and one's descendants was that of
stewardship. This doctrine takes its point of departure from the creation narrative in the book of Genesis.
As this doctrine was developed through the centuries,
it was assumed that this stewardship was exercised in
relation to the limits inherent in the orders of nature
and society, both of which were presumed to be static
and ordained by God. As such, this model suggested that
there were limits inherent in the order of nature and
society and that stewardship suggested both the maintaining of these limits and conformity to them.

In the light of the influence of the theory of
evolution and advances within the science of genetics,
some are suggesting that a more proper description of
human responsibility might be that of co-creator.
Ironically enough, Robert Francoeur locates this
perspective in the same biblical narrative.

> But it seems to me also that in our
> panic we have deliberately avoided one
> of the most basic premises of our Judeo-
> Christian tradition. We have always
> said, often without real belief, that
> we were and are created by God in his
> own image and likeness. "Let us make

man in our image, after our likeness"
logically means that man is by nature
a creator or at least a co-creator in
a very real, awesome manner. Not mere
collaborator, nor administrator, nor
caretaker. By divine command we are
creators. Why, then, should we be
shocked today to learn that we can now
or soon will be able to create the man
of the future? Why should we be horri-
fied an denounce the scientist or
physician for daring to "play God"?
Is it because we have forgotten the
Semitic (bibilical) conception of
creation as God's ongoing collaboration
with man? Creation is our God-given
role, and our task is the ongoing
creation of the yet unfinished, still
evolving nature of man.[14]

This orientation, while containing some overtones
of a promythian presumptiousness, suggests rather that
humans now have the ability to enter into the process of
evolution, to shape it, to direct it, and to redesign
different life forms. As Karl Rahner notes: "He no
longer simply takes stock of himself, but changes himself; he contents himself neither with steering by his
own history merely the alteration of his sphere of existence nor with the mere actualization of those possibilities which have always offered themselves to man in his
commerce with his fellowmen both in peace and in war.
The subject is becoming its own most proper object: man
is becoming his own creator."[15]

The model of co-creator assumes that nature is dynamic and changing and that the end of the process is open, but related to the absolute future of humans. The exercise of responsibility in this model comes about from helping to shape and direct the evolutionary process according to values and criteria that are perceived to be appropriate in the light of goals that will promote human and social good. Given this new state in development as well as a new understanding of nature, the model of co-creator seems at least as appropriate as that of stewardship, if not more appropriate.

Along with this debate on the model through which responsibility should be exercised, there is a continuing debate surrounding the whole understanding of personhood. The discussion centers on both indicators of humanhood as well as on qualities that are appropriate for human beings in the pursuit of their ends and goals. Joseph Fletcher made the initial contribution to the former debate by suggesting a variety of indicators of humanhood which included criteria such as minimal intelligence, self-awareness, self-control, a sense of time in the past and future, a capacity to relate to others, concern for others, communication, control of one's own existence, curiosity, changeability, a balance between rationality and feeling, idiosyncracity and neocortical function.[16] In a later article, Fletcher singled out neocortical function as the essential trait, the key to humans.[17] This is because of the role of the neocortex in providing the biological sine qua non of all human activities. There were a variety of responses to Fletcher's original criteria which were more or less happy with them, depending on one's starting point. Nonetheless, in spite of the somewhat cavalier attitude with which they were proposed, Fletcher did provide a service by pointing to

several problematic areas in defining a human being and
stimulating debate on these problems. Even so, we must
remember that even widely accepted criteria of indicators
of humanhood would not provide the total basis on which
a determination of the value of a human being would rest.

Another contribution towards the understanding of
personhood in terms of desirable qualities is provided
by Alasdair MacIntyre.[18] MacIntyre establishes his criteria not by setting minimal criteria by which one
would be judged to be a person or not, but by arguing
for qualities that would be desirable in designing one's
descendants. These include: an ability to live with
uncertainty, an understanding of one's past which
provides a sense of identity, the ability to engage in
non-manipulative relations, finding a vocation in one's
work, accepting one's death, developing the virtue of
hope and a willingness to take up arms to defend one's
way of life. These are very suggestive elements that
are important for understanding who persons are and how
they relate to others, to society and to nature. The
first quality that MacIntyre suggests, the ability to
live with uncertainty, is a very critical virtue, especially in light of the theory of evolution. It had
previously been thought, and was a deep psychological
consolation, that the orders of nature and society were
stable and normative. They were perceived to be rooted
in an unchanging order of the universe, established
by its creator. For better or worse, we know that this
is not the case, and one of the realities with which
we must make our peace is the fact that our world is
changing and will continue to change. Therefore, the
ability to live with a lack of certainty is a highly
desirable personal quality. MacIntyre very wisely,
however, roots the quality of being able to face an

uncertain future in a sense of identity that comes from
a strong sense of the past, one's place in a family, in
a neighborhood and in a community. Knowledge of self
and one's origins provides the strength needed to face
an uncertain future. Two other of the qualities that
he mentions are very important. The first is the need
to find meaning through one's work. There is a twofold
suggestion here. One is that we need to find meaning
in our lives and one of the places where we can best
find this is through the vocation that we have in the
world. The other dimension is that there are some
things that are worth doing and that it is important that
they be done regardless of their consequences. The
second element that is of importance is the virtue of
hope which is belief in the reality that transcends
what is available as present evidence. The virtue of hope
helps take us beyond a purely rational orientation to
reality and provides us with a larger framework with which
to both see and evaluate what we might be about as we
face our uncertain future.

     Both of these orientations towards understanding
the person suggest important issues. Fletcher, in his
own way, emphasizes the role of rationality and planning
in defining human qualities. In other writings, he has
suggested that the more something conforms to rationality,
the more human it becomes. For Fletcher the use of
genetic engineering, screening programs, amniocentesis
and the like in insuring the birth of a perfect child
is more human because such processes make more use of
rational planning techniques. On the other hand,
MacIntyre looks at broader qualities which appear to
make persons more human. He suggests, by implication,
a stance towards nature which presupposes the rational
but transcends it in a sense of both humility towards

the future as well as a sense of hope that one can remain
in control of the processes that will unfold before us.
Both of these models have their strengths and weaknesses.
Both point to significant dimensions of personal experience
and the sense of the self and both suggest a variety of
relationships towards nature that will be important in
re-evaluating the two senses of responsibility toward the
world described immediately above. In some respects both
of these orientations are departures from the traditional
model of the person found in classical western philosophy and theology with its emphasis on a static nature
within a static world. But they are important because
they suggest and allude to critical dimensions of the
person that were not fully taken into account by the
classical tradition. Thus they are extremely helpful
in elucidating several qualities that will be necessary
to cultivate as we begin to redefine our place within
the world.

Another element in the perception of self is the
articulation of one's relationship to one's descendants. This question, of course, looms large on the
horizon because of our growing perception and experience
of the scarcity of resources. It appears to be the case
that we have already left our descendants an environment
which is damaged and a world which has been depleted of
many of its resources. This is not a very positive
statement about ourselves and even less of one about our
concern for others.

Certainly our descendants, whoever they may be,
will have a number of interests similar to those that we
have. The problem is trying to define the basis on
which those interests should be respected, if at all.
Although utilitarian and contract models may not provide
totally satisfactory resolutions to the problem, both

suggest that one should at least look forward to the future
when calculating total utility or when trying to define
how to act justly. Another approach would suggest that
we know that our descendants will need certain basic
goods and that, therefore, they are entitled to these as
a matter of human rights. The orientation here is not
to harm future generations, rather than promote their well
being. Both of these approaches might suggest that we
should leave our descendants at least as well off as we
are, for in doing so we respect their interests and leave
them the resources necessary for an adequate quality
of life.

My orientation towards this problem will also be
affected by how I see myself in relationship to other
human beings. If, for example, I see myself as a solitary
individual with few links to my neighbors and my community,
then the whole question of responsibility to others has
a less significant place in my ethical calculations. If,
however, I see myself in a community which has come from
other communities and which is producing future communities, then it is more likely that I will be concerned with
the environment that I hand on to my immediate descendants.
These moral connections form the basis for evaluating my
actions in the light of my needs as well as those of my
descendants.

Another framework for analyzing this problem
comes from one's orientation toward the end of the world.
If one adopts a more apocalyptic viewpoint, then the
question of future generations becomes somewhat less
critical because when the end comes, it will come quickly and reality will cease to have significance. The apocalyptic orientation suggests that life may not be as
teleological as we would hope and that while all of us
may have goals and aspirations that we wish to see ful-

filled, ultimately the world ends and we with it. On the
other hand, if one has an eschatological viewpoint which
sees the future as the source of goals and values, then
one can see one's self as building toward a reality that
will come to fruition. In this framework it is important
to build for one's descendants a world that can be lived
in and can be a continuing source of hope. If one views
the future through the apocalyptic lens, the question of
the future is not that important because the end of the
world is the end of significance. In the eschatological
framework, however, what goes on within history and
culture is important and stands in relation to the future
that will, eventually, be reached. In this framework,
the relationship to one's descendants is important and
must be evaluated much more carefully.

      3.   Biology and Behavior. A third important
element is the relationship between our biological structure and our behavior. Such issues although traditional
in their origins, have received a tremendous revival
from the growing perspective of sociobiology and the
sophisticated knowledge we have of genetics.

      The concept of altruistic love, expressed as
either giving one's life for another or in being one's
brother's or sister's keeper, has formed one of the
major pillars of the Western ethical tradition. One of
the suggestions of sociobiology is that perhaps such a
high exercise of altruism is not entirely voluntary and
therefore not responsible on the part of an individual.
Rather, such behavior may be programmed into us by our
genes, and thus our altruism is simply a mechanism of
biological survival rather than an important moral virtue.
A British biologist named B. Haldane suggested the genetic structure of such altruistic behavior when he indicated that he would lay down his life for two brothers

or eight cousins. The reason for that formulation was
that it took that many of each group to achieve a genetic identity to his which would make his own sacrifice
genetically acceptable - i.e., insured the same number
of similar genes to remain in the same gene pool. The
basic implication of such a posture is that one is altruistic towards those who are genetically similar to
me because even if I do not benefit myself, I do benefit those who have genes that are similar to mine.
Therefore, from a biological point of view it makes no
difference whether I survive or they survive, because the
same genes will survive and be present in the gene pool
to replicate themselves.

In the framework of E. O. Wilson, one of the contemporary founders of sociobiology, egoistic behavior is
behavior which guarantees that the genes will in fact
cause copies of themselves to exist; altruistic behavior
is behavior that insures that copies of genes that an
organism contains will survive, although they may be
contained in another organism. These biological definitions of egoism and altruism are then used interchang-
ably with the ethical concepts of selfish and unselfish.
The problem is that a direct translation appears to be
rather difficult. On the one hand, behaviors that we
experience as selfish or unselfish are usually conscious
and the result of an evaluation of consequences. A
strategy for a genetic replication is typically unconscious and therefore not under our control. Also the way
in which the words egoism and altruism are used refers
primarily to actions which affect the gene pool. One
could infer that actions which have no significant im-
pacts on the gene pool must be either egoistic or altruistic or, in value terms, selfish or unselfish.

That, however, does not correspond to our experience.
Therefore we must be aware of such an easy and uncritical translation of biological categories into ethical
categories.[19]

Even though Wilson may not have the translation
of genetic terms into ethical terms that he may wish,
Arthur Caplan argues that there is a point at which such
verifications of biological behavior would be relevant
to ethical theory. He illustrates this by his discussion
of psychological egoism and ethical egoism. The theory
of psychological egoism is a factual theory about human
motivation which claims that persons always try to act
in their best interest. If such a factual theory were
true, Caplan argues that the only reasonable basis for
justified ethical behavior would be a theory of ethical
egoism which argues that morality is a matter of self
interest; that the only acceptable and meaningful ethical
principle is always to act to promote your own individual good as much as possible. A significant part of the
argument for this position would be to determine that
genes both actually cause specific behaviors and that
they are the sole causal agent for them. In addition
to the empirical data that a person would have to gather
to prove this position, one would also need to accept
a great deal of reductionistic theory which has its
own theoretical problems.[20]

Sociobiology also becomes involved in discussions of freedom and moral responsibility, as has already
been suggested in the discussion of altruism. Part of
the problem in this discussion involves the clarification
of the concepts of freedom and determinism. If by freedom is meant a radical freedom in which the person is
bound by no constraints whatsoever, then it is clear
that sociobiology as well as traditional philosophy and

theology would be able to mount a strong case against such a concept. On the other hand, if one accepts a more modest theory of freedom in which choices are possible but only within certain parameters, then sociobiology may not be able to argue as strongly against this as some of its proponents may suggest.

The discussion of freedom must also be related to a discussion of determinism. Again, two extremes can be posed. Hard determinism holds a theory of universal causation which argues that for every effect and event there is a cause and that by definition freedom is incompatible with this perception of reality. From a sociobiological viewpoint, this could mean that each of us is genetically determined and, therefore, subject to irresistible compulsions and coercions and must do what our biology tells us to do. Soft determinism would also hold a theory of universal causation but suggests that some causes originate with human beings and that freedom is compatible with determinism; this is a theory of soft determinism. From a biological perspective, it could be argued that each of us has a set of predispositions within us that can cause us to move in some directions rather than in others, but that no one specific action is totally determined.

A theory of hard determinism rules out a sense of both freedom and moral responsibility. If one cannot control one's actions and if one is simply acting in a preplanned manner, one cannot be responsible for one's actions. On the other hand, it does seem necessary to be able to trace a certain chain of causality in one's actions to be able to assign responsibility for them. If one cannot argue back to a variety of factors that caused one to act in a certain way, one should similarly argue that the individual is not responsible. Human behavior cannot

simply be reduced to a set of biological coordinates.
Such reductionism is contrary to our conscious experience
and does not take into account all of the behaviors which
we attribute to free choice and for which we assume people are morally accountable.   In this perspective, moral
responsibility and freedom are argued for in terms of
the causal efficacy of human intentions and volitions
in relationship to genetic and environmental factors.
Such a theory focuses on self determination rather than
genetic determination.   It attempts to subsume into itself a variety of data from different perspectives arguing, however, that the self is the reality which is
ultimately responsible for what is done and assumes that
responsibility can be justified on the basis of a variety
of causalities operating at different related levels.

        The final topic in this section deals with the
setting of social policies which are based on some concept of justice or equality.   Although a variety of
meanings may be read into these concepts, they have
functioned as primary values in American society and as
the basis upon which many policy decisions have been
made.   The belief that all persons are created equal is
the cornerstone of the American way of life.   Yet over
the past several decades many allegations have been made
about genetic differences between people that would seem
to challenge these values.   There are claims, for
example, that intelligence is related to one's racial
group or that aggressive behavior is related to the
presence of an extra Y chromosome.   Such claims, it is
assumed would make a significant amount of difference
with respect to the social treatment of individuals within these populations.

It needs to be said immediately that a particular social policy does not necessarily follow from a set of empirical facts, whatever they may be. The fact that an individual may belong to a particular group that actually has less genetic potential with respect to a certain level of achievement has no necessary relationship to the specific policy that is directed to that group. Thus, for example, a policy could be articulated that would argue that these individuals need more protection because they have less potential: on the other hand, a policy could also be formulated which states that because these people have less potential, they should simply be ignored.

What would be important, though, is that if it would be the case that certain individuals have a particular genetic potential or lack of potential, that fact, when it is established as a fact, should be taken into account in policy making so that realistic policies and goals can be set. This is simply saying that we should not try to do, much less legislate or mandate, that which we are not capable of doing, whether this be biological or psychological. It is both inappropriate and unjust to devise programs to help individuals reach potentials which they are utterly incapable of achieving. On the other hand, the fact that they might be incapable of reaching a certain potential does not mean that they should be discriminated against, rejected by the society or in other ways ignored in terms of sharing in the basic goods of that society. Facts need to be taken into account in setting policy, but social and cultural values mediate those facts as they are incorporated into policy. Genetics does not provide a totally adequate basis for such a social evaluation.

Sociobiology and other research in genetics does suggest that there may be problems ahead for those who have assumed that the concept of equality of persons means equality in all respects. It is quite clear that people are biologically different and therefore have a vast amount of different potentials. It seems quite clear that the potential of each person is limited by his or her genetic background as well as the environment in which they are raised. The fact that people are un-equal with respect to their potential does not mean that they are unequal with respect to their moral value as individuals and as persons. Such an evaluation of equality is independent of biological and environmental differences. Sociobiology and other research in genetics could provide a useful service by providing information about individuals who may have limited potential so that unreasonable accomplishments would not be expected from them. This could protect these individuals from having unreasonable demands made of them and help eliminate some degree of frustration from their lives. However, the determination of such differences does not and should not jeopardize the unique moral value of these individuals as persons.

IV.   Conclusion

Recent developments in genetics have provided an opportunity to review and re-examine many traditional and thematic principles and concepts in ethics. I have included several of these topics and shown how this new knowledge can help reformulate a concept or challenge a traditional orientation. New discoveries in genetics as well as other areas of the life sciences will continue and new applications and implications of that knowledge will occur. I hope that this presentation has provided a framework for examining these problems as well as suggested some helpful directions in thinking about the resolution of these new ethical dilemmas.

FOOTNOTES

1. Pope John Paul II, Redemptor hominis, 15

2. D. Callahan, "The Moral Career of Genetic Engineering," The Hastings Center Report (April, 1979), 9 and 21.

3. J. Goodfield, Playing God: Genetic Engineering and The Manipulation of Life (New York: Random House, 1977).

4. D. Callahan, "Ethical Responsibility in Science in the Face of Uncertain Consequences," Annals of the New York Academy of Sciences, 265: 2-4.

5. R. McCormick, S.J., "Notes on Moral Theology," Theological Studies (March, 1979, 108-109.

6. K. Rahner, "The Problem of Genetic Manipulation," Theological Investigations IX (New York: Seabury Press, 1975), p. 236.

7. L. Kass, "Making Babies Revisited," The Public Interest (Winter, 1979), 54:41.

8. K. Rahner, "Experiment: Man," Theology Digest (February, 1978), 67.

9. K. Dismukes, "Recombinant DNA: A Proposal for Regulation," The Hastings Center Report (April, 1977) 27.

10. D. Callahan, "Ethical Responsibility," 10.

11. D. H. Smith, "Scientific Knowledge and Forbidden Truths," The Hastings Center Report (December, 1978) 30-35.

12. C. Boorse, "What a Theory of Mental Health Should Be," Journal of the Theory of Social Behavior, 6: 61-84.

13. P. Ramsey, Ethics at the Edges of Life (New Haven: Yale University Press, 1978).

14. R. T. Francoeur, "We Can - We Must: Reflections on the Technological Imperative," Theological Studies (September, 1972), 429.

15. K. Rahner, "Christianity and the 'New Man,'" _Theological Investigations V_ (Baltimore: Helicon Press), p. 135ff.

16. J. Fletcher, "Indicators of Humanhood: A Tentative Profile of Man," _The Hastings Center Report_ (November, 1972), 1ff.

17. Fletcher, "Four Indicators of Humanhood – The Debate Matures," _The Hastings Center Report_ (December, 1974), 4ff.

18. A. MacIntyre, "Seven Traits for the Future," _The Hastings Center Report_ (February, 1979), 5ff.

19. J. B. Schneewind, "Sociobiology, Social Policy and Nirvana," in M.S. Bregory, A. Silvers, and D. Sutch, eds., _Sociobiology and Human Nature_ (San Francisco: Jossey-Bass, 1978), pp. 234ff.

20. A. Caplan, "Genetic Aspects of Human Behavior: Philosophical and Ethical Issues," _The Encyclopedia of Bioethics_ (New York: The Free Press, 1978), Vol. II, p. 541.

THE PROBLEM
OF INTERESTS AND LOYALTIES

Ethical Dilemmas in Obtaining Informed Consent

I.   The Problem

In all professions, the problem of the conflict of interests and loyalties inevitably arises. Eventually all persons must at some time and in some way resolve this dilemma. This common problem of such a conflict is of special importance to the various health professions, especially in the area of research and experimentation. Here such a dilemma will always involve at least two elements - the model of the profession and the research subject. Both of these issues must be taken into account in resolving the potential conflict of interests and loyalties in this situation.

For purposes of clarification, a few working definitions are in order to help set a context for the discussion. As such these suggested definitions are not meant to be exhaustive; they are proposed as indicators to provide a partial background for the proposed analysis.

"Interest" refers to a relation of being concerned with respect to some advantage or disadvantage. When we speak of interests in general, we are referring to concerns, needs, or goals of ours in which we have something at stake. There is an involvement on a personal level with the subject under discussion. The problem of interests becomes compounded when one's interests become vested. Parsons defines these vested interests as follows:

> ...the interests in maintaining the
> gratification involved in an established
> system of role expectation...[1]

Here the notion of interest becomes linked with
an institution and its multi-faceted relations with other
institutions. It then becomes much more difficult to
sort out specific personal interests because they become
merged with the interests inherent in institutional
workings and relations.

"Loyalty" refers to a set of normative values or
ideals of the person or institution which serves as the
basis of ultimate commitment. Loyalties are derived
from membership in a normative class and are, in many
ways, a set of commonly shared values. Loyalties
differ from interests in that loyalties refer to one's
normative ideals rather than to one's actual concerns.
Hopefully one's interests and loyalties would be in harmony, but this is not necessarily the case.

In defining "informed consent" one must carefully
avoid omitting a significant detail or including too
many details. Perhaps a better approach is to indicate
some common themes underlying the concept of informed
consent. Obviously information is one of these for the
intent is that the subject be informed in a meaningful
way of what the experiment is and what may occur during
its course. Included in the act of informing is a discussion of benefits and risks. The element of consent
assures that the subject is voluntarily agreeing to
participate in the research. This would also imply the
right to terminate participation in an experiment at any
point. Ramsey suggests that another needed element is
prudence: "...practical wisdom in the appraisal of
cases and specific situations."[2] This is to emphasize
that the obtaining and giving of informed consent are
never simplistic applications of a definition, but
rather the perception of the situation by both investigator and subject from which emerge loyalty and partner-
ship.[3]

Another important element of informed consent, but one that is difficult to include in a definition, is the reality of power. It is obvious that the researcher has a tremendous amount of power over the subject. This may be due to the researcher's institutional affiliation, professional title, connection with a hospital or university, specialized knowledge, or the class difference that exists between the researcher and the subject. Since subjects are often drawn from lower classes, there is either an actual or perceived power difference between the two.[4] Informed consent can give the subject some countervailing power within the experimental situation. At a minimum level, the obligation and practice of obtaining informed consent say a researcher cannot do whatever he or she wishes and help the subject learn that he or she has rights that must be respected, thus equalizing a potentially unequal situation.[5]

With these themes and Ramsey's caveat in mind, the following DHEW definition of informed consent will be used in the rest of the paper.

> 'Informed consent" means the knowing consent of an individual or his legally authorized representative, so situated as to be able to exercise free power of choice without undue inducement, or any element of force, fraud, deceit, duress, or other forms of constraint or coercion.[6]

Regardless of how we articulate or of how we exemplify it, all agree that progress in medicine and the abolition of disease are positive goods and health a significant value. Implicit in these values, however, is the necessity for research and experimentation on human subjects. Chemotherapy, for example, is one

critical element in the protection and preservation of
health.[7] However, drugs ultimately need to be tested on
humans, for animal trials or mathematical models simply
do not indicate fully how a drug may react on a human
subject. Consequently, at some stage in the development of a new drug, human experimentation becomes a sine
qua non which we recognize and accept as a critical part
of health maintenance.

But, such an acceptance reveals a serious problem:
the need to protect the human subject. Most would subscribe to a general claim that the human is a bearer of
certain rights and dignity which are an intrinsic part
of one's personal nature. And, as such, most would also
generally affirm that there are limits to what one can
do to a consenting or unconsenting subject. The necessity of human experimentation to help promote the value
of health is qualified by the personhood of the subject
and there are religious and ethical arguments that prevent the researcher from doing whatever he or she might
want to do, even though the subject has consented.

The general consequence of such a situation is
the recognition of a need to protect human subjects.
This is stated and argued for in a variety of ways and
codes of ethics, but the general thrust is clear: the
personhood of a subject in some way places limits on
how that subject may be treated. We affirm the value
of health and medical advances, but not to the exclusion or negation of the value of the person.

II.   The Ethical Problem
       The need for the protection of human subjects is
recognized by the various professions that have to do
with health care, experimentation, or other related areas
such as anthropology, psychology, or sociology. Although

it is not necessary to analyze all of these codes of
ethics,[8] some should be presented to give the flavor of
their orientation.

Possibly the strongest of such codes is the
Nuremberg Code of 1946. Coming in the wake of the Nazi
war trials the code particularly emphasized voluntary
consent, the necessity of avoiding unnecessary pain or
mental suffering, and a balancing of risks in proportion
to the humanitarian importance of the experiment.[9] The
1954 World Medical Association Code states:

> The paramount factor in experimentation
> on human beings is the responsibility
> of the research worker and not the will-
> ingness of the person submitting to the
> experiment.[10]

This can have two possible readings. A cynical
one would suggest that the rights of the subjects have
just been placed on the back burner. But the statement
also suggests the ethical demand for the responsible use
of power on the subject by the researcher, for indeed
during the course of the experiment the subject must
trust the researcher to be faithful to the information
given and promises made at the beginning of the experiment. Thus there is a subtle emphasis on the continuing loyalty of the researcher to the subject.

An interesting dilemma is posed by the 1962 Army
regulations on the use of volunteer subjects. The statement reads, in part:

> He must have sufficient understanding of
> the implications of his participation to
> enable him to make an informed decision,
> so far as such knowledge does not com-
> promise the experiment. He will be told
> as much of the nature, duration, and

purpose of the experiment, the method and
means by which it is to be conducted, and
the inconveniences and hazards to be expected, as will not invalidate the results.
He will be fully informed of the effect
upon his health or person which may possibly come from his participation in the
experiment.[11]

These guidelines recognize several areas of
possible conflict - but do not appear to resolve them in
favor of the subject. The rights of the subject seem to
be subordinated to the outcome of the experiment. Also,
there appears to be an unresolved conflict between informing the subject of possible risks to health and
withholding information that may invalidate the experiment.

The 1964 Declaration of Helsinki is a strong
statement on the protection of human subjects. An ad-
vance over the Nuremberg Code is the section on nontherapeutic clinical research which spells out a different orientation from therapeutic research, or as the
Declaration states it, clinical research combined with
professional care. The distinction is an important one
for different values emerge in each situation which
cannot be resolved in the same ways. What may be
extremely risk-ladened in a nontherapeutic situation,
may be the only psssible alternative in a therapeutic
situation. The decision to enter into such a risk-
ladened therapeutic situation cannot be judged by
criteria used to evaluate a nontherapeutic one.

The 1971 "Opinions and Report of the Judicial
Council" of the American Medical Association deals with
the ethical regulation of experimentation under Section II of its Code of Ethics which has to do with the

improvement of medical knowledge and skills. The guidelines list three general principles; the subject must
give voluntary consent; the dangers of each experiment
must be investigated by prior animal experimentation;
and experimentation must be performed under proper medical protection and management.[12] These are followed by
a separate discussion of the ethical requirements for
clinical investigation, either for treatment or for
the accumulation of scientific knowledge. Consent and
protection of the subject from effects of the experiment
are common to both situations. The guidelines stress
the responsibility of the investigator throughout the
procedure. They seem to present no innate ethical
dilemmas, but neither do they explicitly deal with the
problem of what should be done, in the nontherapeutic
context, when knowledge of possible results may either
invalidate or weaken the experiment.

The 1973 Principles of Medical Ethics as applied
to Psychiatry[13] do not specifically mention experimentation. The special focus of this Code of Ethics is the
problem and dilemma of confidentiality. The psychiatrists are referred to the AMA Code of Ethics for a
general statement of ethical regulations dealing with
research. An explicit statement on confidentiality as
it specifically applies to some types of psychological
studies and investigations - other than the admission
that "...materials used in teaching and writing must be
adequately disguised in order to preserve the anonymity
of the individual involved"[14] -- could be helpful in
terms of specifying the requirements of the investigation
and the range of rights of the subject in this situation.

The Code of Ethics of the American Sociological Association offers two general principles which relate to Research.

3.   Every person is entitled to the right of privacy and dignity of treatment. The sociologists must respect these rights.

4.   All research should avoid causing personal harm to subjects.[15]

The code continues, in paragraph five to discuss confidentiality, surely an important topic in sociological investigation. The basic problem here is not the general principles, which are correct enough, but rather with their vagueness. The meaning of the terms are left ambiguous enough to be able to cover a wide variety of situations and therefore possibly skirt the ethical dilemmas. "Right of privacy" and "personal harm" are important concepts, but their significance and usefulness diminish in direct proportion to their vagueness.

The 1973 statement "Ethical Principles in the Conduct of Research with Human Participants" by the American Psychological Association[16] presents some interesting value dilemmas. Paragraphs 3, 4, and 5 all deal with the relationship among informed consent, the obligation of disclosure, and the responsibility of the investigator to protect the subject's dignity. Paragraph 4 states the dilemma most clearly:

4.   Openness and honesty are essential characteristics of the relationship between investigator and research participant. When the methodological requirements of a study necessitate concealment or deception, the investigator is required to insure

> the participant's understanding of
> the reasons for this action and to
> restore the quality of the relation-
> ship with the investigator.[17]

Two basic problems appear at once. First, the
document begs the question of whether concealment or deception are necessary; it glibly assumes they are and
procedes from there. Secondly, the document does not
specify when the participant is to be informed of the
"necessary" deception. If the informing is before
deception, there may be no ethical problems involved;
if the informing is post-factum, there are ethical
problems involved - the violation of the rights of
the subject and negation of the values of openness
and honesty. This situation is problematic at least
and to my mind is an unsatisfactory resolution of the
problem.

Paragraph 5 presents a similar problem in that
it requires the respect for the subject's freedom of
choice, but simultaneously says the researcher may
sometimes have to limit this freedom. The researcher,
then, must take special care to protect the dignity of
the subject. In addition to the repeated problem of
question-begging, a new dimension enters in here:
paternalism. Obviously the researcher is the one who is
making the decision and is the one who decides what is
best for the subject in the light of the needs of the
experiment. This is a serious and unresolved problem in
this code of ethics.

As a result of greater sensitivity to ethical issues inherent in the research situation, a growing concern with the rights of the person, and disclosure of
several problematic, if not totally unethical research
situations and experiments, the Federal Government is in

the process of generating guidelines for the protection
of human subjects in experimental situations. A federal
commission was established for this purpose and had recently submitted recommendations for guidelines on fetal
research which have been approved and promulgated by
DHEW. What is almost more important than whatever final
guidelines will emerge, is the national concern and
debate over the problem of the protection of human subjects. One cannot predict the full effect and lasting
significance of such debate, but a major step forward
has been taken that will provide the basis for further
developments.

Of special importance in the proposed DHEW guidelines of 30 May 1974 is the statement that all research
proposals which place a subject at risk must indicate
that informed consent has been obtained from that
subject and cannot in any way be waived and, in fact,
must be documented. This basically means that all
research proposals, submitted for DHEW funding, which
place subjects at risk must have a section on the ethics
of the research in the protocol itself. This implies
that procedures which might have ethical dilemmas must
be faced and resolved.

A definition of informed consent that the proposed DHEW guidelines offer has been quoted above. The
definition is supplemented by statements which affirm
that full explanation of the material must be given, a
description of risks and benefits must be offered, appropriate alternatives must be disclosed, a declaration
of freedom must be included, and the ability to withdraw
from the experiment at any time must be clearly stated.[18]
One critique raised against these guidelines is the exclusive use of the risk-benefit calculus in evaluating
some of the ethical dilemmas of experimentation. Another

problem may involve the need to separate more clearly
therapeutic from nontherapeutic experimentation - the
distinction could be made clearer. Also, there is need
for the composition of the ethical review board to be
specified lest an unfair power advantage be built into
such boards. The final word has yet to be said concerning these guidelines; but as they stand, they indicate basic areas of concern and situations where value
dilemmas may occur.

All professionals have an interest in their
occupations. They wish to perform well, they want their
work to be important, and they want it to be recognized
and well-received. They too must provide for the neces-
sities of life and, in a highly competitive market, the
competition for a limited amount of money could tend to
bring out high levels of creativity in research proposal
and design - and possibly questionable means of obtaining results.[19]

These all contribute to creating a set of personal interests for a professional, goals or concerns in
which he or she is personally engaged. These personal
interests may link up with social interests and become
magnified. If, for instance, science has a high priority within a society, the energies and finances of that
society go towards promoting science and scientific en-
deavors. Interest groups gather to promote special
projects or to help establish priorities. Interests
become merged and fused; personal interests may become
public interests and public interests may be manipulated
to attain one's private interests.

Many charges of scientists, having manipulated
various interests, have been leveled; within the last
decade science has been the whipping boy for many social
and political problems. Yet, in the main, people esteem

both science and scientists (including physicians and other researchers). H. R. Niebuhr suggests several basic reasons for this esteem: (1) Science has provided good things for us; (2) Science makes predictions that come true; and (3) Scientists have been faithful to us.[20] These reasons are augmented by the feeling that science has used its knowledge:

> ...for the benefit of the whole human
> society and for each individual in it
> as though humanity and the individual
> had a value not derived from their re-
> lations to a nation or a caste, or some
> other special value-center.[21]

Even though this basic confidence is present and operative, some problems appear. The very value of science itself may serve as the problem, for vested interests may develop which may shift values and priorities. Parsons suggests that:

> Collectivity-orientation on the other
> hand converts this 'propensity' (of
> loyalty) into an institutional obliga-
> tion of the role expectation. Then
> whether the actor 'feels like it' or not,
> he is obliged to act in certain ways
> and risk the application of negative
> sanctions if he does not.[22]

This implies that pressures brought to bear by institutions - i.e., universities, research organization, or professional societies - may interject their value preferences between the scientist and his or her work. This is not to suggest that such pressures are necessarily illegitimate or in any way a perversion of genuine research. It is to suggest, however that other interests may enter into the picture and may shift one's perception and priorities.

Insofar as one plays an institutionalized role in interaction with other institution- alized roles, the alternatives for action are presented here in terms of the institu- tional definition of the situation.[23]

H. R. Niebuhr suggests that potential problems exist when science begins to accept uncritically narrow or closed value frameworks such as nationalism or truth as an exclusive end in itself to the detriment of other values such as justice and equality. Such conflict of interest has the potential to weaken the faith and trust we have in science.[24]

There are also a number of potential personal conflicts of interest which should be mentioned. All are aware of the decreasing amount of money available for research, the tightening of the job market, and other pressures in the academic community. Such pressures may cause a person to shift interests or focus on the pro- tection of one's interest by engaging in research whose purpose or methods may be questionable. The extent to which this actually happens is one question; the other question - the potential for it to happen given the nature of the case - cannot be naively ignored. We all know that results are important, and when our interests are at stake, values which are normally important to us may fall by the wayside in the ensuing conflict.[25]

In addition to the fact of professional interests, there is also the fact of professional loyalties. A pro- fessional tends to have a certain standard for action. This may be derived from the code of ethics of a profes- sional society, or from a strong set of convictions of what ought to be done in fulfilling one's role. These codes of moral values give the professional a guide by which actions, priorities, and interests may be evaluated.

H. R. Niebuhr suggests that there are elements
within science itself that may help create a set of
loyalties that can guide one's actions. The first of
these is what he calls a morality of enterprise which
implies that one's commitment is to the service one
performs or the cause which one serves. This type of
commitment to the larger good of one's profession can
help to override a short-term focusing on what could be
exclusively private interests. Secondly, there is the
element of self-examination and self-criticism which is
an attitude of openness towards one's research and its
design, procedure, and evaluation. This social dimension
enhances one's loyalty to values such as honesty and
integrity. Such openness, which is expected in research,
again thwarts a possible tendency to base one's research
on vested interests. The third and fourth dimensions of
morality in science deal with truthtelling within both
the scientific community itself and the human community
at large. Minimumly this would imply a willingness to
have errors brought to light but also implies a willingness to share knowledge gained and to examine the purpose for which it can be used.[26]

These different elements within the nature of the
scientific endeavor reinforce the loyalties of the researcher to certain values and ways of proceeding. They
set forth certain standards and goals. In doing this
they provide an ethical foundation for self-evaluation
and criticism.

In many ways, professional codes of ethics are
specifications of these values which are inherent in
scientific procedures. They function as types of middle
axioms for judging particular cases. In doing this, they
focus the professional's attention on value issues and
value claims so that loyalties and interests can be judged.

Some elements in various codes of ethics -- particularly
but not exclusively, those dealing with biomedical research - are also concerned with values that go beyond
the researcher, but which are obviously related to research. Such values would be concerned with the dignity
and rights of the person who is the subject of the experiment. Although one can easily and correctly argue that
values such as respect for the person, truth-telling, and
respect for privacy are part of the scientific endeavor
itself, it is important that such value claims are also
grounded outside the profession. This clearly separates
the issue of loyalties and interests. When a professional's loyalties transcend a situation at hand, a con--
flict of interest and loyalties can show up more clearly
and has the potential for a more equitable resolution.
What happens, then, is that values impinge on the
professional both from within and without the profession itself. This gives a broader base of support to one's
fidelity to loyalties and has a potential to weaken narrow interest-based claims. A summary statement of the
issue is provided by H. R. Niebuhr:

> ...does not the issue lie between those
> whose good is the collective representa-
> tation of a special group and those who
> trust in and are loyal to the collective
> representation of mankind as a whole?[27]

In a recent article,[28] B. B. Page suggests that
professions open to individuals are not the property of
the individuals in the profession but rather of the
society. Page argues that this is so for two reasons:
(1) "...any individual in any society - even a counter-
culture commune - acquires recognition, relevance and
even meaning primarily in terms of his or her relationships to that society, its culture and institutions,

and its other members."[29]; (2) "...professions acquire
recognition and relevance primarily in terms of the needs,
conditions and traditions of particular societies and
other members."[30]

What this means is that membership in any profession cannot be thought of as separate from one's membership in society. In fact, membership in a profession is
a way of specifying social obligations and responsibilities. Thus, rather than reinforcing a rather tenuous
separation of the individual and society, the fact of
membership in a profession is a way of integrating the
individual and society, in that the profesional has
specific skills to deal with social needs or problems.

Such an understanding of a practice of a profession would go far in helping to resolve, or at least
place in a more significant context, the dilemmas that
can exist between interests and loyalties. First, the
profession is not perceived as being in a conflictual
situation (us against them). Rather, it is one institution among others seeking to contribute to the common
good. It obviously has its own priorities and its own
orientations, but what it has to offer is a contribution
or service of society. Its primary focus is not exclusively its own preservation, but the preservation and
well-being of the society of which it is a member and
which it serves. Secondly, the professional is not simply
a member of a profession. He or she is also a member of
various other civic or voluntary associations. As such,
a professional is, to use Michael Waltzer's phrase, a
"pluralist citizen,"[31] one who shares in ruling and being ruled precisely because of one's multiple membership
in various associations. Each of these associations, to
a greater or lesser degree, proposes various values or
ideals. The internalization of these values is one

additional means of the professional's developing a set
of loyalties which ultimately may transcend the interests
of any single association. Through this process, interests, endemic to only one group, and loyalties, which
transcend any one group are more easily separated and
evaluated. Such a separation of interests and loyalties
does not guarantee more ethical decisions but does contain
a strong potential for forcing professional interests -
vested or not - into the clear light of day to be evaluated
either on their own merits or hopefully, in the light of
one's transcendent loyalties.

The quality of one's ethical decisions may be in
direct relationship to one's degree of specialization.
If a professional becomes increasingly focused on only
one issue and orientation, then there is a corresponding
danger that everything will be evaluated in terms of that
one issue and its interest. This situation obviously
places a professional in opposition to society, for
society consists of more than one issue, need, or
service. If, on the other hand, the professional with
his or her needed and valued specialization - has the
ability to participate at least in an inner dialogue
from a variety of value positions and social viewpoints
which stem from membership in various associations, then
the issue may be resolved more in terms of loyalties to
personal or social values, rather than narrow interest-
based reasons. Such a professional will continually be
in the process of evaluating issues and programs from a
variety of viewpoints with the positive result that
none of these will a priori have the upper hand. In this
situation, loyalties and transcendent values have at
least an equal chance to compete against powerful interest-based reasoning.

As applied specifically to the research or experimental situation, such a framework may be of ethical significance in that it forces the researcher to view his or her work in a wider social perspective, within the context of a variety of loyalties in addition to the specific interests involved. The significance of such a framework is that is casts the ethical dilemmas in research in a context much broader than one determined solely by professional or other interests. Secondly, if a researcher is in this wider context, he or she will have a variety of viewpoints from which to evaluate ethical dilemmas. One will not automatically exclude a set of issues because they do not relate to or bear upon one's own personal or professional interests. Involvement in a variety of associations can also have the beneficial effect of forcing us to entertain a variety of values. And it is this pause for reflection that can induce a greater degree of ethical sensitivity in the research situation. Thirdly, this type of context may cause the process of decision making to be extended. While this is not necessarily a virtue, neither is it intrinsically a vice. In areas where significant value issues are at stake, sometimes an extended period of time is necessary if the full range of values is to be considered. Such a process helps to ensure that interests will not be the sole element in decision making. Interests are significant and need representation; but if they are the only elements that are represented, then a variety of needs and values are always automatically excluded. Such a situation may well produce some short-term experimental benefits; but one also needs to look at the long run. Decisions that incorporate a variety of loyalties and values have the potential to expand one's horizon and to be more critical in the necessary evaluation of consequences, benefits, and risks.

III.   Conclusion

One of the major purposes of this paper is to suggest a new model for understanding a profession. Traditionally, professions have been viewed as specialized groups, quite often far removed from the public and its needs, and concerned primarily with their own interests and goals. Oftentimes, however, this can lead members of the profession into an adversary relation with society (i.e., society may not need or want what the profession has to offer) or into a paternalistic relation with society (the profession'a knowing what is best for society). What this often means in practice is that a profession becomes another interest group, pursuing its own interests without much concern until these interests are challenged and the profession is forced to defend them.

The model suggested here would attempt to broaden the concept of a profession by incorporating wider loyalties into its structure. These wider loyalties, which could come from a professional code of ethics the values or goals of civic, religious, or other voluntary organizations of which one is a member, or one's personal code of ethics, can help the professional realize that he or she cannot define social participation or social responsibility simply from one perspective, i.e., the profession. Other dimensions of life, although perhaps not as dominant as the professional, need to be incorporated into one's modus vivendi so that a pattern of personal and social coherence may emerge. The significance of this model is that it attempts to open up the concept of a profession from within so that the profession may be more easily perceived and defined in relation to and as a part of society - rather than being in an adversary relation. This has the major advantage of helping professionals to understand themselves

as an organic part of a social whole in which a variety
of nonprofessional loyalties must be harmonized with
professional ones.

The wider understanding of a profession is not intended to reject needed specialization, the valued services offered by professions, or the legitimate interests
of a profession. Rather it is suggesting that such
professional services need to be defined to heighten the
relation of the profession to society and to a wider
loyalty base. Such an orientation will not automatically
ensure that more or better ethical decisions will be
made. What this model will do, however, is to intro-
duce into this very concept and model of a profession
value dilemmas that cannot be easily brushed aside. For
if membership in a profession can highlight other social
values and can help in the personal integration of alternate points of view, then the professional will be forced
to become more conscious of his or her multi-faceted
relations with the larger society and the responsibilities that such relations bring with it. By suggesting
that the model of a profession be broadened from within
through the incorporation of a wider loyalty base rather
than accepting a free-market style competition for power,
influence and the attaining of self-defined interests,
there is the posibility that the professional will be
forced to perceive his or her self in a new light and
in a new, more integrated relation with society.

As applied to the informed consent issue, this
framework, simply stated, will help insure that values
other than the interests involved in the research itself-
its methodologies, its claims, and its potential for social
good - be brought to bear on the rights and values of
the subject of the experiment. If the professional conducting the experiment has been involved in a wide
variety of activities, he or she may have been in situa-

tions in which values and loyalties have been proposed from other contexts or persepctives. These values and loyalties will hopefully be integrated within the professional person to produce a moral whole and to serve as a means of testing and evaluating specific interests, which might automatically predispose him or her to act, if not routinely, at least uncritically. Also the paternalism which is quite inherent in a traditional profession may be broken down or weakened. For if the professional is forced to perceive the research subject as a fellow citizen, a degree of equality may be restored to the situation. This in turn will, of course, weaken the power of the professional over the subject. But this is precisely the function of informed consent and the suggested model of a profession may help reestablish the significant role informed consent ought to play in experimentation.

In the issue of informed consent, such a new professional context may, at the least, give the subject an even break; at the most, it will ensure that he or she will be treated with the full dignity due a human being. Since health is a value and since ultimately human subjects are needed for experiments to test products to make or keep individuals healthy (physically or psychologically), it is incumbent upon professionals to separate clearly narrow, profession-based interests from the value inherent in the research situation so that the ethical dilemmas may be clearly stated and the major issues set forth before a final decision is made. Such a model of a profession would enhance the value and significance of the profession itself. But it would do this by incorporating the profession into a wide range of social interests and loyalties rather than by understanding the profession as separate from the community because of narrowly defined interests and loyalties.

FOOTNOTES

1.   Parsons, T: The Social System, The Free Press of
     Glencoe, 1964, p. 492.

2.   Ramsey, R: The Patient as Person, New Haven Yale
     University Press, 1972, p. 3.

3.   Ramsey, op. cit., cf. pp. 5-6.

4.   Cf. Herbert Helman, "The Rights of the Subject in
     Social Research: An Analysis in Terms of Relative
     Power and Legitimacy," American Psychologist
     27: 090-1016, Nov., 1972.

5.   I am grateful to Dr. Dan McGee of Baylor University
     for suggesting this theme to me.

6.   Protection of Human Subjects, DHEW. Federal Register,
     Vol. 39, No. 105, 30 May 1974. p. 18917.

7.   Fuchs VR: Who Shall Live? New York, Basic Books,
     Inc., 1974, p. 30.

8.   For an excellent representative sampling of such
     codes, cf. Henry K. Beecher, Research and the
     Individual. Boston, Little Brown and Co., 1970,
     pp. 217-309.

9.   Ibid., pp. 227-228.

10. Ibid., p. 240.

11. Ibid., pp. 252-253.

12. Opinions and Reports of the Judicial Council.
     American Medical Association, Chicago, 1971, p. 10.

13. "The Principles of Medical Ethics with Annotations
     Especially Applicable to Psychiatry." Reprint
     from American Journal of Psychiatry, September, 1973.

14. Loc. cit.

15. Code of Ethics. American Sociological Association.
     Reprint from the American Sociological Association.

16. American Psychologist, January, 1973, pp. 79-80.

17. Loc. cit.

18. Federal Register, op.cit., p. 18917.

19. Barber, B., Lally, J.J., Maharahka, J.L., et al:
     "The Structures of Scientific Competition and
     Reward and its Consequences for Ethical Practice
     in Biomedical Research." Paper presented at the
     67th annual meeting of the American Sociological
     Association, 1972. Cf. also, by the same authors,
     Research on Human Subjects: Problems of Social
     Control in Medical Experimentation. New York,
     Russell Sage Foundation, 1973.

20. Niebuhr , H.R.: Radical Monotheism and Western
     Culture, New York, Harper and Brothers, 1960,
     pp.79-80.

21. Ibid., p. 81.

22. Parsons, op. cit., p. 98.

23. Parsons, T.: Essays in Sociological Theory.
     New York, The Free Press, 1967, p. 145.

24. Niebuhr, op. cit., pp. 82-83.

25. Barber, et al., op. cit.

26. Ibid., pp. 132-135.

27. Ibid., p. 88.

28. Page, B.B.: "Who Owns the Professions?" Hastings
     Center Report, October, 1975, pp. 7-8.

29. Ibid., p. 7.

30. Loc. cit.

31. Walzer, M.: Obligations: Essays on Disobedience
     War and Citizenship. Cambridge, Harvard University
     Press, 1970, p. 218.

THE PHYSICIAN—PATIENT RELATIONSHIP

A Shift in Understanding

I always find it both threatening but intriguing
when I read an article that challenges my own frame of
reference but also proposes arguments with which I am at
least half way sympathetic. The New England Journal of
Medicine published a posthumous address by Dr. Franz
Inglefinger in which he discussed his own reaction to the
diagnosis of cancer that he received.[1] Since the cancer
occurred in the area of the intestine in which Dr. Inglefinger was a specialist, he described himself as probably
the ideally informed patient. Yet when it came time to
decide whether or not to receive chemotherapy, what kind
of chemotherapy to receive or whether or not to follow
up the chemotherapy with radiation, Dr. Inglefinger found
himself terribly confused. This confusion was not helped
by the advice that he received from his daughter and son-
in-law, both of whom were physicians, nor from the many
physicians around the country who sent him their advice.
Dr. Inglefinger only experienced some relief from his
confusion and information overload when he listened to
the advice of a friend who told him that what he needed
was a doctor. Once in the care of a competent physician,
Inglefinger listened to his advice, followed it, and was
comforted by the course of treatment prescribed for him.

Such an anecdote about a morally sensitive and well-
informed physician does much to argue against the current
wisdom that patients must be informed as fully as possible
about their disease before they can make an informed decision about the treatment strategy. One could infer from

his story that if such a well-informed physician was
overwhelmed by the choices to be made, what hope does
the ordinary and obviously less informed citizen have
when it is his or her turn to make such a complicated
and awesome decision.

But the moral of this story may not focus on
autonomy and consent as much as it does on the quality
of the physician-patient relationship. I would like to
address the physician-patient relationship by discussing various models of the relationship and some directions for the future.

I will first describe four images of the physician
proposed by Robert Veatch.[2] Second, I will present
three models of the physician-patient relationship developed by Szasz and Hollende.[3] Third, I will discuss the social context in which these images and relationships occur. Finally, I will present my conclusions.

The first model of the physician is that of the
engineer or technician. Here the physician is seen primarily as a scientist, focusing on the disease process,
divorcing himself from consideration of personal issues,
and especially divorcing himself from any value issues.
The physician is a technician whose values and ethical
orientation are subservient to the facts of the situation and decisions are made exclusively on the basis of
those facts.

I do not think that this model addresses the
general practitioner, the family physician, or individuals involved in some form of primary health care. It
is a model, however, that is relevant for the sub-
specialist or tertiary health care provider. Typically
in those situations the patient has been referred to
the specialist and the specialist's role is perceived
to be to diagnose and remedy, if possible, a particular

problem and not necessarily deal with the patient as a whole. Thus, while this model may not be appropriate for the majority of situations in which a physician might find his or herself, nonetheless it may be applicable in a particular situation or for a particular purpose.

The second model is the priestly model which is derived from the feeling that the physician has power over life and death. The physician is seen as a quasi priest because he or she defines criteria for human behavior, criteria for risk taking and, in fact is influential in helping people become better. The powers of the physician become augmented because of the responsibility that he or she has for caring for human beings and because of the esteem in which most people of most cultures hold a physician. This model provides the physician with a wide range of authority and decision making and, while in this model the physician may typically follow the traditional Hippocratic duty of doing no harm, it is the physician who defines what harm is, what harms may be appropriate or necessary.

This model frequently finds its way into common perceptions of a physician, at least implicitly if not explicitly. The model becomes most critical when a physician helps a person recover from a serious illness or when a physician makes an accurate diagnosis that provides the way out of a particular problematic situation. The issue here is more a function of how the physician is perceived rather than a desire of the physician to accrue power to his or herself. A physician, I would think, should always be wary of how much a perception of his or her stature can influence the relationship -- for good or bad.

The third model is the collegial model in which
the physician attempts to be the friend of the patient
who is then encouraged to work in harmony with the
physician as colleagues pursuing a common goal. The
physician, in this model, is to identify with the
interests of the patient and adapt to the values and
background of the patient so that they can build up a
common bond of trust and loyalty. In this model the
physician, as in the model of the engineer or technician,
is to discount his or her own values and attend only to
the values and interests of the patient. In this way the
patient is given the proper dominance in the relationship
and has his or her own needs responded to and protected.

While there are some attractive features to this
model, it assumes that the values, concerns, and professional skills of the physician are not that critical
to the interaction that is occurring. Such a model
carries with it the danger that the physician must
continually compromise his or her own values and respond only to what the patient perceives as good for him
or herself. On the other hand the model does suggest that
the patient has his or her own values and interests and
that these must be attended to in determining what is to
be done.

The final model is the contractual or fiduciary
model. This is not to be understood as a strictly legal
contract, but rather as a relationship in which there are
reciprocal obligations and duties. This relationship is
based on mutual trust and confidence, even though there
is not and will not be a full mutuality of interests or
values. This model attempts to encourage the development
of a context in which both the physician and patient can
state what is important to them, what the problems are,
and on what interests and values they will base their
decisions of what is to be done.

This model allows both the physician and patient to maintain their own integrity as they attempt to search for a common resolution of what is to be done. The model also allows each member of the relationship to exercise their proper responsibility. This model may not make decision making any easier, but it does have the benefit of arguing that responsibility for decision making is not the exclusive prerogative of either the physician or the patient.

Another way of looking at the physician-patient relationship is in terms of the modes of interaction between the physician and patient. While these descriptions will somewhat overlap with the models I have previously described, they nonetheless provide a different way of thinking about the relationship.

The first mode of interactivity is activity-passivity. In this model the physician is the actor, the one who is doing something, the one who has control over the situation. The patient is passive, is the recipient, and follows out the orders of the physician. The prototype of this mode of interaction is parent and child. There are extremely important and appropriate clinical applications of this model in an emergency, when a patient is in a coma, or when a patient has suffered a severe trauma. Here the patient can do nothing but be passive and receive the care of the physician and the physician must be active, must take control.

The second mode of interaction is that of guidance-cooperation. In this mode, the physician is perceived as an authority and as the one who will perform a service for a patient, but within limits. The patient must cooperate with the physician to receive the full range of benefits but also must be informed enough to take control

over certain areas of his or her life. The prototype of
this relationship is parent and adolescent. This suggests
that while the parent has authority and control, the
adolescent is also beginning to emerge from a position
of being controlled to defining his or her own sense of self
and is assuming more self-control. The clinical application of this model is that of a serious illness or an
infectious disease in which the physician's effectiveness
is defined by the actions of the patient.

The final model is that of mutual participation.
In this mode, the physician's goal is to help the patient
help him or herself. The patient is seen as a partner,
as one who must assume more and more control and responsibility for his or her own state of health. In this
mode the roles and expectations of each are more clearly
defined and cooperation proceeds on that level and with
that understanding. The prototype of this relationship
is adult to adult in which the relationship consists of
two adults each of whom has his or her own interests and value
and who are brought together to attempt to resolve a
particular problem. The expectation here is that each
will use the appropriate skills and responsibility to
achieve that goal. The clinical application of this relationship is a chronic illness, psychoanalysis, or
chronic heart disease.

What I think is important in each description
of these modes of interaction is that there is an appropriate clinical setting for each mode. Thus, as I
mentioned, in an emergency the physician must be active
and the patient is, by definition, totally passive.
If one is in analysis or has a chronic disease such as
hypertension, one would assume that the physician would
attempt to help the patient develop strategies to deal
with life situations that are problematic with respect

to the condition. The physician cannot live the patient's life; the patient must be led and encouraged to do this for his or herself; ultimately, to assume responsibility for his or her health. Conversely, it is inappropriate to assume that a patient will be able to assume responsibility for his or her care during an emergency. Here the physician must be active and must assume control so that appropriate medical interventions can be made to benefit the patient.

Describing these modes of interaction can be helpful with respect to helping physicians and patients understand different ways of interacting and to determine which may be appropriate in a particular situation. As I mentioned, the problem comes not from a physician's assuming control of a situation or providing needed advice, but when the physician or patient assumes that there is only one way of interacting and that this is normative for all situations.

Having described these different models and modes of relating to patients, let me now more thematically address the issue of the social forces which have brought about a change in the physician-patient relationship as traditionally understood, and articulate some of the issues that are involved in that. Again, the models and modes of interaction that I have described will be a reference point for this discussion.

The traditional model of the physician-patient relationship was quite clearly understood and, in fact, was sanctioned by both physicians and patients. The patient described the problem to a physician who listened to what was said, asked questions, made a diagnosis, and gave orders that the patient was to follow. The patient then accepted these orders and at least occasionally did what the physician said.

While this description of the traditional physician-patient relationship may be stereotypic, it nonetheless contains many truths. The physician played a
very active role and the patient tended to play a very
passive role. The role of the physician was to give
orders with the assumption that the patient would follow them. The physician was perceived as having the
means, if not the power, to cure a particular disease,
whereas the patient was perceived as powerless and not
having the ability always to understand what was happening to him or her. In this traditional model, the only
recourse that a patient had, if he or she disagreed with
the physician, was simply to go to another physician.
Challenging the authority of a physician was something
that was simply not done. The traditional model thus
reflected parent-child interactions and a priestly model,
and occasionally the engineering model.

Then, a new social force arose, beginning in the
late 1950's, which had a significant impact on the traditional model of the physician-patient relationship.
This new social force was the "rights" movement, beginning with civil rights for blacks and followed closely
by the Women's Rights Movement, the Children's Rights
Movement, the Gay Rights Movement, and the Consumer's
Rights Movement.

This social phenomenon has had its impact on the
physician-patient relationship, and the traditional
model is beginning to change. A variety of court cases
have opened up the relationship for a closer scrutiny
than ever before, and some physicians feel that many of
their medical judgements are improperly being challenged by non-physicians. Others feel that the rights
movement is reducing their role to that of a technical
advisor and is further jeopardizing an already tenuous

relationship with the patient. Finally, many feel that
the Consumer's Rights Movement is, at least by implication, casting aspersions on the physicians' motives and
interests in treating a patient. Such orientations clearly signify a loss of autonomy for the physician, but
more important they also strike at the physician's self
image, and thus, too, the physician-patient relationship.
Therefore, although many physicians may in general be
open to the rights movement and renegotiation of the
physician-patient relationship they are nonetheless very
dismayed by their perception of the reformers' motives.

On the other hand, many patients, although they
may be aware of the Consumer's Rights Movement, are
themselves extremely uncomfortable about assuming the
new, more participatory role that is the natural outcome of the rights movement. Because of the widespread
acceptance and affirmation of the traditional passive
role of the patient, many patients may simply be unpre-
pared to assume responsibility for their medical management. Others may feel inadequate to help in the decision making process in terms of devising a treatment
regimen that is in harmony with their life style priorities. Still others may simply not wish to accept this
responsibility at all. "Doctor, what would you do in
my situation?" may still be the most common response
that many patients have when a physician asks them for
their input during the decision making process.

What will probably be the case then is that until
the newly emerging model of physician-patient relation,
which is fiduciary and parent-adolescent or adult-
adult, becomes clarified both parties will feel quite
threatened by what they are asked to do or not to do.
But even though this transitional period may be problematic for many persons, it is extremely important to

remember that a participatory type of physician-patient
relationship allows two very essential things to happen.
First, the physician can continue to exercise the traditional role of patient advisor and, in fact, this
dimension of the physician's role might be enhanced.
Second, the values that are important to the patient
can more easily and quickly come to the surface.

One implication of the participatory or fiduciary
model is that it will encourage physicians to look beyond an exclusively clinical evaluation of a patient's
medical problem in an attempt to understand it in the
context of the patient's life situation. This model
encourages the physician to know the patient as a person, giving him or her a better perspective of who the
patient is, what the patient does and why, and what impact the patient's actions and life style may have on
his or her health. This broader understanding of the
patient will allow a physician to make more relevant
suggestions to the patient in terms of what he or she
can do to enhance his or her health and to prevent further recurrence of illness. But more important, the
physician can also gain that very important "sense of
the person" that is extremely critical to his or her
role as an advisor of the patient. Within this model,
the patient will know that the physician is open and
receptive to what he or she says, will know that the
physician is interested in more than "just the facts,"
and that the physician will indeed lend an appropriately
sympathetic ear when needed. The model allows both to
be active and to assume appropriate levels of responsibility.

The participatory model of decision making will
also allow patients to state, either implicitly or explicitly, the values and priorities that they have in life.

Often enough, many medical problems and the treatments
recommended for them have a considerable impact on a
person's life style or occupational goals. Questions
of the benefits vs. risks of treatment, life style implications, and cost are immediately raised. Although a
patient may want to be cured, he or she may also be quite
resistant to changing behavior or to rearranging priorities to help effect that cure. A patient may, therefore,
reject medical care, not because he or she thinks the
physician is wrong, but because he or she simply does not
want to adjust priorities or values to fit the treatment
regimen. The primary discussion in this situation thus
centers on not the medical facts per se, but what those
facts mean for the patient.

Let me now return to the anecdote about Dr. Inglefinger as a way of summarizing different elements I think
appropriate for the relation between the physician and
patient. I argue that the relationship should be a fiduciary one. This kind of relationship is characterized
by high levels of trust and openness to the clearly stated
values of each member of the relationship. In such a
fiduciary relationship, both partners can be respectful
of the other's values, although the patient more often
than not may be willing to be led by the judgment of the
physician as articulated in treatment decisions. In
this type of a relationship, the physician focuses on
the good of the patient, assumes the role of advising
the patient, and accepts a high degree of responsibility
for the patient's best interests. This orientation
neither diminishes the role of the patient nor ignores
the patient's values. Rather, the patient assumes that
the physician can see beyond the narrow interests of the
patient to what might be overall in the best interest of
the patient, from both a medical perspective as well as

from the perspective of the person's life project. The patient's autonomy and competence are complimented by the physician's care and loyalty to the patient. The fiduciary, adult-adult model has the potential of combining the best aspect of autonomy and personal value of each, without surrendering to a destructive individualism which puts both in an adversarial relation.

In a fiduciary relationship, a physician will be paternalistic and authoritarian, but not in a way that demeans the patient or ignores his or her values or occupational goals. Such a relationship allows the physician to have unique insights into the patient and to have a sense of his or her interests, as well as an understanding of the person's values and what they mean to that person. Such information and insight is valuable in helping to ascertain the competence of the patient and what limits of responsibility he or she is comfortable with at this time. And while this kind of a relationship is not always possible, it nonetheless provides a model for the kind of relationship that is most helpful in understanding the interests of a patient. Such an orientation helps the physician to avoid an uncritical paternalism and helps him or her to recognize the limits of autonomy that each of us experience, especially when we are ill. The fiduciary model of the physician-patient relationship allows the physician to go beyond a narrow contractual or legalistic model and enter into a significant, personal relationship with the patient and, on the basis of this relationship, to help the patient articulate what is appropriate with respect to his or her care.

With the possibilities for disagreement that are latent in the participatory or fiduciary model of the physician-patient relationship, significant issues for both physician and patient will quickly come to the surface and receive the attention they so desperately need. What is of genuine importance to each party can be discussed in a more open manner and each can be more sensitive to the concerns of the other. Of course, this type of relationship is also more complicated, more time consuming, and much more demanding on the physician as well as the patient. The participatory of fiduciary model can only complicate the already complex life of a busy and responsible physician, as well as place further demands on the patient. Nonetheless, if such a participatory or fiduciary model is accepted and practiced by the physician and patients it is likely that both will be more open, receptivity to medical and personal advice will be more easily given and accepted. In such a relationship, therefore, each will be exercising appropriate responsibility and the goal of the relationship -- the restoration to health of the patient -- can be more easily and ethically attained.

FOOTNOTES

1. Franz Inglefinger, M.D. The New England Journal
    of Medicine. 25 December 1980.

2. Robert Veatch. "Models for Ethical Medicine in a
    Revolutionary Age." The Hastings Center Report.
    2 (June 1972), pp. 5-7

3. Thomas S. Szasz and Marc H. Hollende. "The Basic
    Models of the Doctor-Patient Relationship,"
    Archives in Internal Medicine, 97 (1956): 585-592.

THE WITHDRAWAL OF TREATMENT

The Costs and Benefits of Guidelines

The Karen Ann Quinlan case, and the multileveled
tragedies that followed in its wake, focused national
and international attention on a problem partially caused
by the very technology designed to resolve it: the
treatment and care of individuals in a terminal illness
or in irreversible coma. Technological advances have made
it possible either to maintain physical life or to prolong dying almost endlessly. Unfortunately these advances have not been as effective in providing a cure
or restoring such patients to an adequate level of
health. Given this situation, many are questioning the
wisdom of continuing treatment when no reasonable benefits are to be expected, while others question the ethics
of not doing all that is possible.

Because of this ethical and medical dilemma, and
as a result of a suggestion by the New Jersey Supreme
Court, some institutions are turning to the use of
"Ethics Committees" (Teel, 1975) whose responsibility
is to determine whether there is a reasonable hope of
the individual's ever returning to a cognitive, sapient
state and, thus, to help decide whether to employ life-
prolonging technology. The acceptance of such committees
as the appropriate mechanism for dealing with the comatose patient is apparent from the number of guidelines
for the evaluation of such patients that have recently
been published - guidelines that include recommendations
for terminating treatment if medically appropriate.

The Purpose of this article is to review the guidelines proposed by Beth Israel Hospital, the Massachusetts General Hospital, Mount Sinai Hospital, and several New Jersey medical associations. While not wishing to suggest that these are the only guidelines available, I have chosen these particular documents for examination because they have all been recently published, they discuss a variety of issues, and they raise certain ethical problems. Consequently, they serve as a good point of departure for discussion the issues and problems surrounding such committees.

I.   The Beth Israel Guidelines

The Beth Israel document (Rabkin, 1976), is the most general, dealing as it does with patient-physician decision making, and not exclusively with the intensive care unit. The document evolved from the Law and Ethics Working Group of a faculty seminar on the Analysis of Health and Medical Practice - an activity of the Center for the Analysis of Health Practice of the Harvard School of Public Health. Although two attorneys and one physician authored the article describing the guidelines, neither the names nor the professional status of the other participants is mentioned. At present this proposal is not actual policy at Beth Israel, although consideration is being given to using it as such.

The proposed Beth Israel guidelines are based on three general principles: (1) that the general policy of hospitals is to act affirmatively to preserve the life of all patients, including patients who suffer from irreversible, terminal illness; (2) that hospitals are to respect the competent patient's informed acceptance or rejection of treatment; and (3) that regardless of the hospital's prolife policy, the right of a patient to decline medical procedures must be respected.

A variety of approaches are proposed to help deal with the problems that emerge as a terminal illness progresses. "When it appears that a patient is irreversibly and irreparably ill, and death seems imminent, the question of the appropriateness of cardiopulminary resuscitation in the event of sudden cessation of vital functions may be considered by the patient's physician, if not already raised by the patient, to avoid an unnecessary abuse of the patient's presumed reliance on the physician and hospital for the continuation of life-supporting care." (Rabkin, 1976) Implied in the statement is the belief that although the patient comes to the hospital for treatment and consents to the procedure, it is nonetheless appropriate to test this consent at different stages of an illness to attempt to balance the interests, rights, and duties of both the hospital and the patient.

When the illness appears to be irreversible, then a medical evaluation and a diagnosis is made by the responsible physician. But any decision to withhold resuscitation becomes effective only upon the informed choice and consent of the competent patient. In this context, competence refers to the understanding of the relevent risks and alternatives, as well as a deliberate choice of the course to be pursued. The physician is cautioned to ensure that consent does not come from a temporary distortion because of pain or medication. Also, if the physician feels that the patient is not able to deal with making such a decision at this time, resuscitative efforts must be employed. Once the patient chooses, his or her choice may not be overridden by the staff or the family. Permission to inform the family must also be obtained from the patient and his or her instructions must be followed.

If the patient is incompetent, the final decision for orders not to resuscitate must be based on a
concern for the patient's point of view; the focus for
such a decision must be the clinical interest of the
patient. No other factors can be considered because
this would violate a fundamental prolife policy of
the hospital. A final condition for the issuance of
orders not to resuscitate an incompetent patient is the
approval of the same family members who are required to
consent to a postmortem examination.

The Beth Israel document stresses that orders not
to resuscitate a patient do not imply any intent to
diminish appropriate medical and nursing attention
needed by the patient. It emphasizes that every effort
must be made to provide a level of comfort and reas-
surance which is appropriate to the patient's state of
consciousness and emotional condition, regardless of
any designation of incompetence. The document concludes with a notice that any request not to resuscitate
that originates from members of the family is not to
be viewed as the patient's choice. Thus the attending
physician and any committee involved in the decision-
making process must not simply concur with the family's
request, but should go through the procedures suggested
above.

Several positive elements in the proposal need
to be emphasized. First, it is an attempt to respond to
the host of problems caused both by the complexities
associated with a terminal illness and by the limits of
technological intervention. Second, it implies that
economic considerations not be the sole criterion by which
decisions to terminate resuscitaion measures are to be
evaluated. Third, the document attempts to deal with the
potential legal problems raised by the decision to

terminate treatment. This is not done crassly to avoid
a malpractice suit, but is a responsible effort to address problems that have been raised in the past. Fourth,
the patient is the center of attention in that the
patient is recognized as the ultimate decision maker.
Finally, the document is respectful of the patient's
decision, even to the point of arguing that if the
physician finds the "...medical program as ordered by
the patient so inconsistent with his own medical judgment
as to be incompatible with his continuing as the responsible physician, he may attempt to transfer the care of
the patient to another physician more sympathetic to the
patient's desires." (Rabkin 1976) This is also exemplified by the statement that the competent patient's decision
may not be overridden by the family and that they are to
be informed of it only after receiving the patient's permission to do so.

Two major problems, however, are created by the
stipulation that physicians may unilaterally order resuscitation for those competent patients who they feel are
psychologically incapable of participating in critical
treatment decisions. The first problem revolves around
establishing the criteria for evaluating whether a
patient is able to cope with such decision making. The
only criterion mentioned in the Beth Israel document is
reasonable and humane medical practice, which, unfortunately, is vague and not subject to review. Consequently, this can open the way to possible abuse of the
patient's presumed reliance on the hospital and physician
for continued life support care. The second problem is
that since neither the patient nor the family has given
consent, the resuscitation effort constitutes treatment
without consent and therefore is an assault on the
patient. While one would not like to see critically ill

patients treated cruelly or unfeelingly in the name of honesty and autonomy, neither is it appropriate to deny patients opportunities for giving or refusing consent in the name of humanity or reasonable medical practice. Indeed, such is not even medical practice; it is the unwarranted imposition of a possibly alien set of values on another.

Another problem arises with the ad hoc committee which determines "whether the patient's death is so certain and so imminent that resuscitation in the event of sudden cessation of vital function would serve no purpose." (Rabkin, 1976) The problem is not that there is such a committee, but with its membership and status. The committee is to be composed of the attending physician and nurses and one staff member not previously in the patient's care. Such membership can easily lead to a biased discussion of the patient. The majority of the members may be locked into a preference for a certain therapy and thus may not discuss the full range of options. Also, the vested interests of the various professions may preclude an unbiased discussion of the situation. If the patient is competent and is given the opportunity to make decisions, such a committee is unnecessary. Also, in the case of a comatose patient, it is unclear who has the responsibility for convening such a committee. Nor is it clear, in this case, that a committee decision not to resuscitate can take precedence over the substitute consent of the next of kin. In the document, approval of the committee's decision by the next of kin is required. Such approval is obviously necessary; but it is unclear why the family's decision is only that of approval. Given a prognosis, it seems proper to allow the comatose patient's next of kin to make the decision since they may possibly know the patient's values, interests,

and preferences better than the medical staff. Although
problems may possibly arise here also, since the legal
status of the next of kin is uncertain in this situation,
this approach seems preferable to attempting to dis-
guise a value judgment as a medical one.

II.   The Mount Sinai Guidelines

Other guidelines for dealing specifically with
patients in intensive care units have been established.
One example, that has been in practice for 5 years now,
is the informal patient-care classification system in use
at the Falk Surgical-Respiratory Intensive Care Unit of
the New York Mount Sinai Hospital. (Kirchner, 1976) Four
levels of care have been established: (1) all-out
therapeutic effort; (2) continuation of all-out effort,
but with 24 hour revaluation of the patient's prognosis;
(3) conservative, passive care, with no heroic measures
to prolong life; and (4) all therapy and life-support
assistance discontinued for brain-dead patients (based
on the Harvard Ad Hoc Committee's definition of death).

This classification system was born out of staff
frustration arising from the use of heroic measures which
seemed merely to prolong dying and from the lack of a
mechanism for reaching a consensus on how to treat critically ill patients. The system, however, is an informal one and has never been presented formally to the
hospital administration. Also the treatment category
number never appears on the patient's chart - only on
the charge nurse's record sheet. Finally the classification system is not routinely explained to attending
physicians. Each patient's status is reviewed every
morning on unit rounds and if the staff decides a
change in classification is indicated, this is discussed
with the attending physician. If the attending physi--
cian should want a change, this is discussed at after-

noon rounds and, if possible, a decision is made that same day. The head of the intensive care unit has final responsibility for decision making, but if any members of the team insist that maximal therapy be continued, it is.

Two major problems emerge with the practice described here. First, the team does not involve the family in the decision-making process. "Rather," according to the current director of the intensive care unit, "it's a matter of asking them to accept the doctor's decision." (Kirchner, 1976) The team keeps the family informed about the prognosis and the therapy being used; no change in therapy is made without the family's knowledge; and if the family wants to keep a terminally ill patient alive as long as possible, the team does so. However, the family is basically presented with a fait accompli. Since no routine explanation of the classification is given to the physician, one can hardly expect that such an explanation is given to the family. Also the decision to terminate treatment is a value judgment based on a medical prognosis, but this distinction is fatally blurred by the decision-making methodology.

The second and more critical problem is revealed in three sentences from the article reporting this system. "Patients with every chance of survival often beg the staff to stop treatment, but naturally, nobody takes them at their word. 'All they really want is relief from constant pain and anxiety,' says Diane Adler. 'We give them more pain relievers and spend more time talking with them.'" (Kirchner, 1976) The problem words here are "naturally" and "really wants." Why is it natural that no one listens to the patients' requests? It is because they present an alternative

value system or is it because their desires contradict
what the staff thinks is best for them? Also, since no
one listens to patients, how does anyone know what they
really want? Patients indeed may want relief from pain
and anxiety, but they may also want something else and
they have the right to be heard and have their competent
decisions carried out. Despite the argument that
patients are usually too sick to participate in the
decision-making process, the exclusion of competent
patients from this process results in treatment without
consent. Such treatment is legally an assault, as well
as a questionable ethical practice.

In the intensive care unit, treatment decisions
must often be made quickly and hence guidelines such as
these could be helpful in assessing the available options.
However, the purposeful elimination of the competent
patient and the family from the decision-making process
is a serious defect in these guidelines.

III.   The Massachusetts General Guidelines

A subcommittee of the Critical Care Committee of
the Massachusetts General Hospital in Boston has developed a set of guidelines similar to those at Mount Sinai.
(Critical Care Committee, 1976) Although the four levels
of patient classification are practically identical,
several significant improvements have been introduced.
First, the guidelines have been accepted by the hospital's
General Executive Committee, the highest medical-policy
committee in the hospital, thus giving the criteria
official recognition. Second, there is an Optimal Care
Committee available to all intensive care units and
other physicians who request advice in the management
of therapies. This committee provides the opportunity
for the case to be reviewed by someone who is not directly
involved in it and thus has the potential for widening

the basis of decision making. Third, the guidelines require that "appropriate notes specifically describing
the therapeutic plan should be made on the patient's
record." (Critical Care Committee, 1976)

In spite of these improvements, the Massachusetts General document contains three critical problems.
The first is that the attending physician makes the
final decision about treatment regardless of what the
Optimal Care Committee or staff may say. This raises two
major problems. The first deals with consent, which is
not discussed in the document. If the patient is competent, any decision about treatment is properly the
patient's; if the patient is incompetent, the authority
to give proxy consent should fall to the next of kin.
The other problem is that the centering of authority in
the physician confuses medical and value judgments in
therapy. The physician is the proper one to make a
prognosis, but a variety of values enters into the
implementation or rejection of the therapy and these
values may not be the ones the physician would choose.
Such confusion gives unfortunate support to the fic-
tion that medicine is value free and further weakens
efforts to obtain the consent of the patient or the
next of kin.

A further shortcoming stems from the fact that
the guidelines are management oriented. While not
wrong - and in fact quite necessary - this orientation
nonetheless leads to an emphasis on the procedures by
which information is communicated between the physician
and staff and the procedures by which the physician's
decision is implemented. This makes the patient even
more marginal to the decision-making process and even
more a totally passive recipient of the medical care
delivery system. An exaggerated emphasis on the

management of the patient to achieve consensus on his
or her treatment can lead to effectively neglecting the
interests of the patient.

The third deficiency is the failure to provide
clearly defined criteria for reaching treatment decisions.
For example, when a patient is reclassified as Class C
(selective limitation of therapeutic measures), he or
she is to be transfered out of the intensive care unit
and "certain procedures may cease to be justifiable and
become contraindicated." (Critical Care Committee, 1976)
The reclassification decision is to be based on the
needs of the patient and only after required comfort
measures become manageable in a nonintensive care setting. Unfortunately, the criteria for evaluating the
patient's needs and the appropriateness of various procedures are not discussed. The assumption is that they
are medical, value free, and presumably self-evident.
While it may be quite proper to limit treatment selec-
tively, this is not totally a medical decision and
ought to be based on more than vague references to
patient needs. The failure to designate who is to make
this sort of decision and the lack of clear criteria
for making it are serious lacunae.

In summary, the omission of a discussion on
consent, the centering of authority on the attending
physician, and the lack of criteria for decision making
severely weaken the usefulness of the Massachusetts
General Hospital guidelines.

IV.   New Jersey Medical Associations' Guidelines

Another orientation to some of these problems is
provided by guidelines designed by three medical societies
in New Jersey. (State Medical Society, 1977) These guidelines are a specific attempt to implement the New Jersey
Supreme Court's ruling in the Quinlan case that an

"Ethics Committee" be used to evaluate the attending physician's judgment that no hope of restoration to cognitive, sapient life exists. If such a committee agrees with the physician, life-supporting measures may be removed without criminal or civil liability. This committee, designated as a prognosis committee by the guidelines, is selected by the responsible governing authority of the hospital or other facility. Membership is to include representatives of standard medical disciplines plus any specialist who may be needed for a particular case. At least two nonstaff members should be on the committee; a physician of the family's choice may consult with the committee and attend its deliberations. The attending physicians are specifically excluded from the committee. The committee may be activated by either the attending physician or the patient's family or guardian. The committee is to review the patient's record, seek other medical information as necessary, and examine the patient. After a clear consensus is reached, the committee shall report as to whether there is a reasonable possibility of the patient's ever emerging from the comatose state to a cognitive, sapient state. This recommendation shall be part of the patient's medical record.

Of the several advantages of these guidelines, the first is the clear recognition that the committee's task is to make prognoses, not decisions regarding termination of treatment. The mandate of the committee is narrowly defined and this helps to clarify the different aspects of the decision to terminate treatment. Second, the attending physician may not be part of the committee. This both removes potential conflicts of interest and provides for independent review and evaluation. Third, the guidelines are clear on when and how the committee

is to be activated.   This procedural point is missing
in the other documents even though it is crucial for the
initiation of a review.

The major problem with these guidelines is best
illustrated by the following excerpt from the guidelines:
"The attending physician, guided by the committee's decision and with the concurrence of the family, may then
proceed with the appropriate course of action and, if indicated, shall personally withdraw life support systems."
(State Medical Committee, 1977) This provision reduces
the role of the family or guardian to one of consultation rather than primary responsibility. The early part
of this same paragraph recognizes that the committee's
responsibility in evaluating a prognosis is limited to
the application of specialized medical knowledge to the
case. The above quoted, concluding sentence confuses the
distinction between medical and nonmedical decisions and
assumes that the attending physician is the appropriate
one to make both types of decisions. Such generalization
of expertise is basically fallacious and also serves to
take the responsibility of decision making away from the
family or guardian where, according to the New Jersey
Supreme Court, it belongs. (In Re Karen Quinlan, 1976)
Thus, while the guidelines follow one suggestion of the
court, they ignore an important requirement of the court.

V.   Unresolved Problems in Intensive Care

The medical and ethical dilemmas raised in the
treatment of the terminally ill are serious and difficult.
It seems that no matter which way one moves, problems
emerge which further frustrate all parties. Therefore
the remainder of this article is devoted to discerning
the thematic connections among these problems and discussing their implications for the development and use of
guidelines for critical care.

The most critical issue is that of patient competency. It is clear, legally and ethically, that the competent patient has the right to refuse any treatment. Given this, many of the provisions in the guidelines discussed above are useless because they assume that treatment decisions are within the scope of the physician's authority. This preempting of the patient's right needs to be more seriously addressed by the medical profession than it is here. For if the patient is competent and makes his or her decision, the guidelines are not needed.

The incompetent patient presents a variation on the consent for treatment theme. The central problem is determining who can give consent for the incompetent patient. Traditionally parents have been allowed to give consent for minors. With respect to the incompetent adult, a legally appointed guardian of the person may make decisions regarding the individual's physical status and bodily integrity. Usually a spouse or other next of kin can make these decisions, although the legal status of their authority is somewhat unclear. A mechanism for circumventing the proxy consent question has been introduced in California, where state statutes now allow competent adults to issue legally binding instructions regarding the treatment to be given them should they become incompetent. In the Quinlan decision, the New Jersey Supreme Court argued that third parties (i.e., guardians or next of kin) can exercise the incompetent patient's right of privacy, a right which includes the prerogative of terminating treatment. It is quite unclear why the guidelines exclude these people from the decision making process. For the most part, the guidelines designate the physician as the proper decision maker with respect to the termination of treatment, a decision which does not turn solely on medical factors. Yet the physician is typically not the parent, spouse, next of kin, or legally appointed guardian. Since the rationale for this situation is not given, one can only infer that the working assumption is that the one best qualified to make the technical decision is also the one best qualified to make the ethical or value judgment. This patently fallacious generalization of expertise is common to all of the guidelines and represents their most critical weakness.

The second theme concerns the management of the patient and staff. In such a critical area as the the intensive care unit, where decisions with extensive consequence must often be made quickly, it is most important to have clear procedures for decision making. Confusion and conflict serve no good purpose generally and, in an intensive care unit, they can literally be fatal. Yet with respect to guidelines for strengthening this process, the question of whom they are to benefit must be raised. Are they to enhance the treatment and care of the patient? Or, are they to reduce the tension and guilt associated with such decisions by artificially creating a show of unity and consensus behind which hide all sorts of unresolved problems among the staff? It should be kept in mind that the staff is there for the patient, not vice versa. The Massachusetts General Hospital document in particular focuses on the benefits accruing to the attending physician in terms of increased support from and reduced conflicts within the staff. But such a management goal is achieved only at the cost of ignoring the patient. Guidelines that attempt to incorporate different points of view have many procedural problems; those that resolve problems by disregarding critical elements have many legal and ethical problems.

Unfortunately, some elements of the guidelines discussed here tend toward the latter.

The third major issue (which is not addressed by any of the guidelines discussed) is the question of who will ensure that the officially accepted guidelines will be followed. Unfortunately, it is much easier to develop guidelines demonstrating one's legal and ethical concern for the patient than it is to follow through on implementing the guidelines and dealing with all of the problems and tensions they inevitably raise. While wishing neither to burden anyone with further committee responsibility nor to establish yet another committee, I must note that it is imperative that steps be taken to ensure that patients and families are informed of treatment guidelines, that the staff follows them, and that changes in policy or interpretations of policy are brought to the highest authority in the hospital for approval.

The fourth theme is that of economics. Although only the Massachusetts General Hospital guidelines explicitly reject economics as the sole criterion for decision making, this rejection is implicit in the other guidelines as well. In these days of the increasing use of cost-benefit and cost-effectivenss analysis in health policy, as well as escalating costs for medical care, such a rejection provides a solid measure of comfort. It indicates that the primary concern is the patient and his or her welfare. Yet, one can wonder if other types of quasieconomical decisions, such as the allocation of scarce resources (e.g., ICU beds), are not being made continually. If they are, the criteria for such decisions should be clearly stated and fully explained to the patient, staff, and family. The rejection of economic criteria narrowly defined as ability to pay seems to be a reasonable element in any guidelines and one that might

be fairly easily agreed upon. The resource allocation
decision, however, presents ethical, economic, and medical problems and will not lend itself to easy consensus.
Nonetheless, this element of decision making must be
clearly incorporated into treatment guidelines because
of its far-reaching implications.

Finally, one can raise the ultimate question of
the necessity of such guidelines at all. The right of
the competent patient to refuse any treatment is well
established. (Annas, 1977) At best the guidelines are
superfluous in this situation. They have strategic
value in that they reinforce this basic legal and ethical
right; they give nothing new to the patient, however.

Regarding the incompetent patient, other issues
arise with respect to who shall make the decision to
terminate treatment. The first is that this is not
entirely a medical decision. Although it is initiated
by medical judgment, it is fundamentally a value,
religious, or ethical decision. Hence; the physician-
qua-physician should not be the primary decision maker;
rather, the guardian or next of kin should be given this
role since they have been charged with serving the
interests of their wards. This was emphasized in the
Quinlan case where the argument was made that third
parties can exercise the right of privacy on behalf of
their wards. Also, as "living wills" become more legally
acceptable, the patient may already have made his or
her decision with respect to treatment, thus removing the
need for guidelines specifying the decision makers.

With respect to the content of the decision made
by guardians, Veatch makes two helpful suggestions. The
first is that a refusal of life-saving treatment is unreasonable if the treatment would restore reasonably
normal health to the patient. The second is that it is
not unreasonable to reject death-prolonging treatment

(Veatch, 1976) This view implies that treatment guidelines should be primarily concerned with establishing a
mechanism by which guardians can obtain accurate long-
range prognoses. The orientation of the guidelines,
however, seems to be that of giving the physician the
criteria for decisions regarding treatment. The New
Jersey guidelines are somewhat of an exception for they
recognize that the function of the committee is to clarify and/or confirm a prognosis. But, even here, the
physician is the one to determine whether treatment should
be continued. The implication is that the guardian or
next of kin only consents to the decision of the physician. Unfortunately, the correct process is the reverse.

It is my contention that treatment guidelines are
useful only insofar as they serve to clarify the prognosis
and likely outcomes of various treatments so that the
guardian and next of kin can make an informed decision.
In their present form, then, the guidelines falsely serve
to legitimize the physician as both the chief decision
maker and the one who specifies the content of the decision. When this authority is restored to those to whom
it rightfully belongs - the guardians and/or next of kin -
then the guidelines will serve the more proper function
of defining the medical status of the patient and the
outcomes of various therapies.

The growing development and availability of
sophisticated instrumentation in the intensive care unit
has brought us to a keen awareness of the limitations of
medical technology. Because such machines can serve to
prolong dying as often as they serve to restore health,
hospitals have developed guidelines to help in the decision making process. As long as such guidelines serve

as a means of generating information for competent patients, guardians, or next of kin to make the best decision they can, the guidelines are useful. But if they serve to validate the status quo of removing such decisions from the responsible parties and reserving it to the physician or staff, they overstep their own proper role and work against the patient and his or her own interests and values.

BIBLIOGRAPHY

1. Annas, G.J., (1975). The Rights of Hospital
    Patients. New York: Avon Books (79-91).

2. Critical Care Committee (1976). Optimum Care for
    Hopelessly Ill Patients. New England Journal of
    Medicine 295(7): 362-364, 12 August 1976.

3. In Re Karen Quinlan: An Alleged Incompetent
    (1976) 355 A 2d 647.

4. Kirchner, M. (1976). How Far to Go Prolonging
    Life: One Hospital's System. Medical Economics:
    12 July 1976

5. Rabkin, M.T.; Gillerman, G.; and Rice, N.R. (1976)
    Orders Not To Resuscitate. New England Journal of
    Medicine 295(7) 364-366, 12 August 1976.

6. State Medical Society (1977). Guidelines for Health
    Care Facilities to Improvement Procedures Concerning
    the Care of Comatose Non-Cognitive Patients.
    January 1977.

7. Teel, K. (1975). The Physician's Dilemma: A
    Doctor's View: What the Law Should Be. Baylor Law
    Review 27(1): 6-9.

8. Veatch, R.M., (1076). Death, Dying, and the Biological
    Revolution: Our Last Quest for Responsibility.
    New Haven: Yale University Press, (162).

DYING IN A TECHNOLOGICAL AGE

I.   A Triumph of Technology

Much more than the fictional dictatorship of the computer "Hal" in the movie 2001, the trial of Karen Quinlan may well have revealed something of the real relation between humans and technology. Indeed, the decision that Ms. Quinlan must be artificially maintained by her respirator may be a clear signal that humans stand in a new relation to technology and the products of a technological civilization.

Humanity has spent the last few centuries rejoicing in its freedom from the domination by the powers of nature. Now it may suddenly find its position reversed. Only this time the dependency may be a creature of humanity's own making. One reason for this is because of what many have called the "technological imperative." Simply stated, this means that if we can do it, we should do it. In many ways this imperative lies close to the heart of America for it stresses the virtues of pragmatism, activism and capitalism. But if it is allowed to operate uncritically, we may find that it will bring us closer to the science-fiction fantasies of the totally technological society.

Of all the many questions that have been raised by the Quinlan case, the question of the technological imperative may be the most important, for it sets forth the basic ethical and social context in which all other questions have to be asked. However, it is the imperative itself that needs critical evaluation. In many ways, it has been a working hypothesis of contemporary society

and of health care in particular. While technology may
be forcing ethics to re-evaluate some of its principles
and conclusions, ethics must also force such a re-evaluation of the basic premises of technology so that the
values can be clearly stated and their operational consequences can be evaluated.

The principle of the technological imperative is
extremely critical in the Quinlan matter for it shapes
almost preconsciously our feelings and value-responses
about the situation. If it is evident that we can continue to maintain Ms. Quinlan on a respirator almost indefinitely - and there is the technological capacity to
do so - then who are her parents, or anyone else for that
matter, to demand that the machine be turned off? What
right do we have to terminate what technology can prolong?

What has happened in this process is a subtle -
but extremely critical - reversal of the traditional
question about the use of extraordinary or heroic means
of treatment. Traditionally, the ethical task has been
to justify the use of extraordinary means of therapy or
treatment. In the usual ethical interpretation, extraordinary has meant very expensive, experimental, or
medicine proper to the disease, but which is incapable
of restoring the person to health. The principle has
always recognized that what is extraordinary can become
ordinary; but it still clings to the test of the potential for restoring health for evaluating the treatment.
Pius XII - no flaming liberal - argued that one was
never obligated to use such means even though death would
certainly and knowingly follow. The basic reason is
that the ethical tradition saw people as bound to use only
what would be ordinarily required to maintain health.
And, at least in the Catholic tradition, there is the
recognition that life is not the highest value and that,

therefore, one is not obligated to do what is extraordinary to preserve it. From this framework, one can
fairly easily argue that Ms. Quinlan need not be maintained on the respirator. It is an extremely expensive
procedure and on that basis alone very extraordinary.
Also the treatment - including the use of the respirator -
has no potential to restore her to health. It is very
important to recognize that there have been no medical
claims that she will ever be cured or restored to a
meaningful degree of health, even though her physical
life may be maintained.

However, an extremely important shift seems to
have taken place. A working presupposition of many connected with the trial seems to have been the preservation
of life for its own sake. The major reason for this may
be that we now have the technological capacity to prolong life almost indefinitely. The question has been
moved from whether we should turn the machine on to
whether we should turn it off. The problem of whether
this treatment may be extraordinary or beneficial seems
to have vanished. Very little emphasis is being placed
on whether Ms. Quinlan's treatment may have any benefits
to her - other than artificially maintaining her at a
rather low level of even physical existence, to say nothing of the quality of her personal life. Part of the
reason for this shift in orientation may be the simple
presence of the machines in the hospitals. We have
them and therefore we use them. Another reason may be
that such technological advances represent a way of
avoiding our embarrassment over death, for we now have
a way to put off this final affront to modern medicine.
A final reason may be the uncritical and unexamined acceptance of such technological advances as an unquali-
fied good. We have designed the machines; they work

exceptionally well; therefore they and their effects must be good. When stated in such a form, the technological imperative is easily recognized as illogical. But when disguised as modern medical care and treatment, it may not appear in this unfavorable light. But however one interprets this major shift in the ethical analysis of such cases, there must be an evaluation, for a shift such as this is too important an issue to enter our lives uncritically.

A triumph of technology will occur if the technological imperative is not brought forward and clearly examined. But this most basic question was not called into question at the trial. The problem of active vs. passive euthanasia, the degree of control humans have over their own lives and the lives of others, the specter of a renewal of Nazi-type atrocities, and the Vatican's last desperate grasp at control over the destiny of individuals all pale in comparison to the problem of determining whether we ought to do all that we can. To make such a decision uncritically or on the basis of some false issues raised in the Quinlan case would be the greatest of follies and the most unethical of all possibilities.

The Quinlan case represents an important crossroad for humanity. For the decision that the machine should not be turned off may mean that we are entering a new age and will find ourselves in a new relation to technology. If the right to terminate such treatment had been upheld, humanity would have been affirmed as the master of the technology it designs, rather than its servant. As it is, the fate of Ms. Quinlan may reveal much about ourselves and our future.

II.   The Court's Verdict

As has often happened during the course of the
past year, Karen Quinlan hauntingly smiles at us from the
front pages. This time the story says that the New Jersey Supreme Court decided her father may seek a physician
willing to stop the respirator which has ruthlessly kept
her from death for over a year. Now that it is clear
that no further legal maneuvers will be attempted, this
decision should be the penultimate chapter in one of
the major tragedies of modern medical practice.

Even though the case may end mercifully with
Ms. Quinlan's death, some issues have been raised by the
Court which merit further investigation and evaluation.
This case is by no means unique and developments within
medicine and medical technology will continue. Continued
reflection seems to be imperative.

Based on the published reports of the new decision, the Court saw value in some issues posed by ethical
commentators, although these issues are properly articulated within a legal and medical perspective. One note
of comfort in the decision is that physicians now distinguish between curing the ill and comforting the dying.
Implicit in this is the recognition that while there is
an obligation to cure the ill, there may be an obligation
only to care for and comfort the dying. The Court said
such attitudes are balanced efforts to implement a proper
respect for the meaning of life and death. While I personally laud the Court for accepting this position, I
also think it is a shame that this viewpoint, a tradition of Roman Catholic medical ethics and a principle
well developed by Ramsey in 1970, has taken so long to
sink into the consciousness of many and to be legally
implemented.

The recognition of the Court that the act of turning off the respirator is not an act of either criminal or unlawful homicide is also a positive sign. There is a clear recognition that the cause of death will be the failure of the biological processes to maintain themselves - not the removal of the respirator. Put in much simpler terms, one can argue that the Court recognized that, in common experience, all of us will die - regardless of the quality or quantity of various holding actions or medical machines. The Court properly distinguished between the unlawful taking of the life of another and a certain amount of self-determination in the act of dying and asserted that the recognition of death's inevitability hardly infers the right to murder. Such a distinction clearly removes this discussion from the categories of active or direct euthanasia and places it within the human experience of death as the fate of us all.

A third encouraging note is the Court's recognition that there comes a time when individual rights overcome the State's interests. The clear suggestion is that the closer individuals come to their death, the weaker State's interests over them become. While applauding this conclusion with its clear implication of some kind of right to be left alone, one needs to raise the issue of exactly what the State's interest is. How far into one's life can the State reach? How is the value of life enhanced socially and individually by artificially maintaining the biological processes of unconscious dying patients? One may ask if the interest of the State may not better be articulated in terms of protecting the citizen from uncritical application of technology which may have the capacity to stabilize or maintain persons while neither curing them nor restoring them to reasonable health. We need to recognize that there is a real

problem in adapting either too casual or too strict an
approach to medical care; yet within this dilemma, the
interests of the State with respect to the individual
must be clearly enunciated and firmly argued. Hoisting
the flag of State's interests may stop a particular action, but in itself does not resolve the issue.

In spite of these generally positive elements in
the recent Quinlan decision, there are also two very
problematic issues. One is the published report of the
gratuitous dismissal of the issue of religious freedom.
The Court relied on the old saw that the right to religious beliefs is absolute, but that religious actions are
subject to governmental restraint. While it is absolutely
clear that the use of extraordinary or heroic treatment
is a moral option within Roman Catholicism, it is by no
means self-evident that the forcing of extraordinary
treatment on individuals is not a violation of their
religious freedom. It is one thing to say that the
public interest is at stake; it is quite another matter
to prove it. Also, since a Constitutional right is
under discussion, all presumptions should favor that
established right, unless clearly stated and strongly
demonstrated vested state interests are brought forward -
and they were not. Much more careful thought needs to
go into the famous distinction between religious belief
and action than is evidenced here. The distinction is
more hypothetical than real. Secondly, the distinction
begs the question of the relation of belief and action
by implicitly suggesting that religious acts - even if
optional - are only tenuously related to religious beliefs and may therefore be impeded without any violation
of First Amendment rights. Finally, the decision fails
to take into account the basic rejection of the Reynold's
principle of separation of beliefs and actions in recent

cases such as <u>Macintosh</u> (1970) and <u>Yoder</u> (1972). The issue of religious freedom in such cases is a profoundly
serious one to which the courts have not been very sympathetic. The time has come for a thorough re-evaluation
of this issue.

The second problematic issue in this decision is
that of the Constitutional right of privacy. Quite properly the Court argues that this right is broad enough
to cover a decision to decline medical treatment under
certain conditions. This ultimate sanctuary of the person appears to be one of the best Constitutional and ethical places to develop a strong argument for this position. The unfortunate part is that the decision did not
stop there; it went on to say that the right to privacy
is broad enough to cover this decision, just as it is
broad enough to cover a woman's decision to terminate her
pregnancy under certain conditions. The problem here is
not necessarily a substantive one. However, it is profoundly strategic.

One of the problems in the discussion of Ms.
Quinlan's situation has been the lumping together of all
sorts of unrelated issues, which has served only to further obfuscate an already murky situation. The Court has
opened itself unnecessarily to the possibility of a strong
attack by extreme right-to-life groups who argue a moral
domino theory with respect to the practice of abortion
and euthanasia. Many expressed relief at the first
Quinlan decision because it was perceived as a way of
stopping euthanasia-on-demand. Now the Court - from this
particular perspective - has not only apparently waffled
on the euthanasia issue, but has done so by using the
same reasons which justify abortion. While neither a
necessary nor a correct reading of the decision, many
may argue that this is the clear implication of it.

Unfortunate as this may be, the ensuing unclarity and hostility will be the fault of the insensitive wording of the decision. Some will always be ideologically incapable of separating issues, but there is no good reason why these groups should be handed such opportunities on a silver platter.

Even though it is an obvious improvement over the first decision in its affirmation that removing a person from a respirator is basically not an act of criminal or unlawful homicide, and in its recognition of the distinction between caring and curing, nonetheless this most recent decision does raise some serious issues that need further investigation. The relation between optional religious actions, religious freedom and forces medication merits much more careful treatment than they have received in the literature and in court decisions. Also the proper relations - and the lack thereof - between the right to life, the right to privacy, and abortion, and euthanasia need to be clearly stated with sound ethical and empirical reasoning. (This material originally appeared in different form in Commonweal /5 December 1975 and 7 May 1976/ and is reprinted with their permission.)

WITHHOLDING TREATMENT FROM NEWBORNS

Complications in Decision-Making

The media continually report stories on newborns
who are allowed to die because of physical and social
problems they present at birth. Baby Doe, who died in
April of this year, had unconnected intestines which made
oral feeding impossible. A simple surgical procedure
can correct that problem. But, because Baby Doe also
had Down's Syndrome - a genetic abnormality causing mental retardation - his parents refused any surgery.
This decision was sanctioned by the Supreme Court of
Indiana and Baby Doe died within six days.

Another case, reported earlier this year,
focused on a rare but tragic complication. Parents in
Illinois gave birth to Siamese twins who were incomp-
letely formed, resulting in children with separate heads,
arms and chests, but joined together at the pelvis,
sharing a common leg. Again, in this case, the parents
refused treatment on behalf of the children and requested they not be fed. Eventually the parents were charged
with attempted homicide, but were not convicted. The
infants received food and medical care and survived.

These are dramatic cases, the ones receiving
national attention. But cases like this occur daily in
the relative privacy of the newborn nursery. Yet these
decisions are becoming more public and an increasing number of medical, ethical, and legal experts are addressing
the problems these decisions present. Also, parents appear to be more assertive in the decision-making process. There is a growing concensus that there are circumstances in which refusal or withdrawal of treatment

is justified. This is most apparent in instances of
severe brain damage, resulting occasionally in an almost total lack of development of the brain, multiple
handicaps which prevent response to therapy, or very
early prematurity.

While not the typical outcome of birth, such
tragedies happen often enough that specialized nurseries-
neonatal intensive care units - have been developed and
are staffed by new specialists including but not limited
to pediatricians, neurologists, psychiatrists, nurses,
social workers. New teams of developmental interven-
tionists provide continual medical and developmental
support to infants, who - appropriately enough - are
said to have "survived."

Yet these individual and team resources are
frequently inadequate - for there is a limit to the
support that can be given to newborns who lack critical
organs or who have multiple defects. Often parents refuse the resources available to their child because they
realize the limits of these resources in restoring their
child to health, because they do not feel capable of
raising such a child, or because they perceive that the
child, even with the best of available medical care,
will have an apparently poor or minimal quality of life.
Some parents do not want a damaged child, regardless of
what can be done.

Physicians and nurses will often support the
decision of the parents, but they also may not. The
way information about the child is presented can
determine how the parents decide. Value judgements
are continually being made, but frequently under the
guise of hospital policy or medical judgement. These
decisions seem to be a bit easier to make when they can
be described as something other than what they actually

are: value judgements, ethical decisions, assessments
of quality of life, or the acknowledgement of personal
prejudices.

Whatever their origin, though, more and more people seem to be deciding to forego treating their newborns
in the hope that they die quietly and mercifully.

The response to this fact or perception of
fact is varied, of course. Some individuals have very
cogently argued that such a practice is severe neglect
of physicians' and parents' obligation to provide a
minimal standard of care for those for whom they are
responsible. Such neglect of duty - evidenced by refusing appropriate medical treatment or food which results in the death of a child - is a criminal homicide.
Others use justice to prevent taking into account
irrelevant issues. If two infants are born with
the somewhat common problem of blocked intestines but one
also has Down's Syndrome, many would argue that justice
is violated if the former is treated but not the latter.
Mental retardation, these individuals argue, does not
diminish the value of the person and, therefore, is not
a morally relevant difference on which treatment could
be refused. Finally, some argue that all of life is
valuable and must be preserved regardless of circumstances. Considerations of the quality of life have no
part in the treatment decision.

Thus the issues are joined: right to life vs.
quality of life; duty to care vs. feelings of inadequacy;
technical ability to maintain vs. responsibility of long
term care; medical prognosis vs. value judgements; hospital policy vs. individual decisions; law vs. conscience.
The purpose of this article is to present a Directive
from the Department of Health and Human Services (HHS),
report several observations on it by Norman Fost,[1] and

draw conclusions on the basis of which I make several recommendations. On 18 May 1982, HHS issued a "Notice to Health Care Providers" on discrimination against the handicapped by withholding treatment or nourishment. This directive is significant because of its direct impact on hospitals, staff, parents, attorneys, and advocacy groups. But the directive will be problematic more because of unclarity than anything else.

This notice, issued by the Director of the Office of Civil Rights, applies sections of the Rehabilitation Act of 1973 to newborn infants suffering from some handicap - mental or physical. One problematic section of the Directive is:

> Under Section 504 it is unlawful for a
> recipient of Federal financial assistance
> to withhold from a handicapped infant
> nutritional sustenance or medical or sur-
> gical treatment required to correct a life-
> threatening condition, if:
> (1) the withholding is based on the fact
>   that the infant is handicapped; and
> (2) the handicap does not render the treat-
>   ment or nutritional sustenance medically
>   contraindicated.

The first problem with the Directive is that it is precisely because the infant is handicapped that discussions about treatment refusal or sustenance denial are initiated. If there were no handicap, such questions would not be raised. But more to the point of the Directive, are there no handicaps that never justify not treating an infant? And, if there are handicaps that do justify non-treatment, is it not the handicap itself that is the primary justification for such a decision? While evaluations of technical feasibility are also important

here, the handicap itself is the focal point of decisions
not to treat. Such tragedies of infants with serious and
multiple traumas present the clearest example of a handicap's justifying not treating the child. What are we to
make of the Directive in the light of this? Does it mean
that all are to be treated as extensively as possible
for as long as possible? Does it mean that if some test
or procedure is omitted that the hospital, staff or parents are liable to criminal prosecution? Significant
clarification is necessary here.

Section (1) of the Directive ignores the reality
that the handicap itself frequently justifies withholding treatment. Although clearly there is much room for
significant debate on which handicaps may justify non-
treatment or the withdrawal of initiated treatment, some
handicaps constitute an insurmountable barrier to life
and, therefore, justify non-treatment.

Section (2) raises another problem, perhaps one
of the most complex ones in medicine. This section
states that the handicap does not render the treatment
or nutritional sustenance medically contraindicated.
There are at least two problems with this statement.

First, what is the definition of "medically
contraindicated"? Several are possible: no treatment
is available at the present time; experimental drugs or
interventions are being developed but their results are
uncertain; effective treatments or procedures are not
available in this facility; effective treatments or
procedures exist and are available, but the person's
condition is so bad that they will not help; the physician doesn't think the available procedures will improve the quality of life of the patient; the parents
don't want the child treated.

Since the Directive provides no definition, we really cannot determine what actually is "medically contraindicated". Clearly, it makes little sense to legislate that physicians shouldn't do what they are not competent to do, should use what is not available, or should not do what is useless. It is clear that it is medically contraindicated to feed orally a child whose intestines are blocked because the child will be further stressed and his or her situation will be worse. If this is all the Directive means, it is not helpful because this definition is self-evident.

But "medically contraindicated" may be a way of attempting to camouflage a second element: the attempt to transform a value judgment into a scientific or medical one. In this case, a decision to withhold treatment is made either on quality of life grounds, feelings of inadequacy on the part of the parents, or a rejection of the child because of the defect. Then that value decision is justified by describing it as a medical decision. Much doubletalk is involved in this, and medical data and risk-benefit analyses may be stretched beyond what is reasonable. But however done, the effect is the same: the value judgment - no matter how well or poorly argued - is improperly hidden under the blanket of "Medically contraindicated."

Thus the first problem that the Directive presents in section (2) is that it either states the self-evident and is trivial or, in a much more serious fashion, will force individuals to go underground with their value decisions regarding treatments by hiding them in medical and scientific terminology. Such encouragement of deception can only make the situation of the handicapped worse off, will encourage physicians to deny the clearly value-ladened nature of their profession, and may encourage parents to abdicate their responsibility for decision-making

The second problem with this section is in its application: how do we know when the handicap renders the treatment contraindicated? The problem here is how to overcome section (1) which says that treatment or food may not be denied because the infant is handicapped. On the one hand, handicaps may not be taken into account and, on the other hand, they may signal a medical contraindication. This situation indicates, I think, both the confusion of the Directive and the complexity of the situation. Apparently there are handicaps which could serve as medical contraindications, but the Directive neither tells us what these are nor provides criteria for assessing handicaps. Such confusion can only bring serious harm to all involved - infant, parents, and staff. The Directive provides no frame of reference whereby parents and staff can work out a resolution and the vague - if not contradictory - nature of the Directive provides grist for many different mills.

By simultaneously affirming what it denies - that handicaps can be a justification for treatment denial - the Directive only contributes to the tragic situation often found in the newborn nursery. Confusion, anger, frustration, and prolonged anguish can be the only outcome of this part of the Directive.

The Directive then goes on to specify three areas that facilities should review to ensure that they do not engage in or encourage discriminatory practices.

> Counseling of parents should not discriminate by encouraging parents to make decisions, which, if made by the health care provider, would be discriminatory under Section 504.

Health care providers should not aid a
decision by the infant's parents or
guardian to withhold treatment or nourishment discriminatorily by allowing the
infant to remain in the institution.

Health care providers are responsible for
the conduct of physicians with respect to
cases administered through their facilities.

This last directive states nothing new whatsoever.
A facility which employs professional staff is responsible
for their actions. Perhaps this will encourage facilities
to develop clear and published policies or procedures on
which administrators and staff agree so that the basic
ground rules don't have to be negotiated for each case.
It goes without saying that these policies should be discussed with the parents. Frequently this can be done
before birth, especially if the mother is in a high-risk
category and is already in dialogue with the staff of
the newborn intensive care unit. Not all problems of a
particular newborn can be discussed before birth and certainly the presence of a baby with serious problems creates
severe emotional trauma that may change one's perspective
significantly. Nonetheless, having discussed the policy
of the facility, having considered various options, and,
more importantly, having established some relation with
the staff may help everyone work their way through
these problems.

The first directive - the staff should not encourage parents to make a discriminatory decision - rightly
argues that the facility should not surrender its appropriate role in decision-making - nor should its staff.
One way out of decision-making dilemmas is for the staff
to abandon the parents by telling them that all decisions

are theirs and the staff simply implements the parent's
wishes. Another way out, implied in the Directive, is
for the staff to provide only one option - treatment -
but make the parents feel that it's really their decision.

The primary problem here is the one first discussed - how, on the basis of criteria proposed in the
Directive, does one know that the staff is discriminating
or encouraging discrimination? No help is provided here.
This lack of clarity can contribute to mistrust among
staff and conflict between staff and family. If there
is no agreement on what is discriminatory, then any act,
however benign, is potentially discriminatory. The directive clearly puts the facility and the staff on notice -
but for what is unclear.

Finally, the directive mandates, in the second
guideline, that facilities may not assist in parent's
discriminatory judgments by allowing the infant to
remain in the facility while not being treated or fed.
Clearly this is one way to solve problems. The attending physician or appropriate administrator simply says,
"OK, Mom and Dad, if you don't want us to take care of
your baby properly, you take your baby home and do it
yourself." Few, if any parents, would have the courage
or strength to do that. Moreover, one can hardly think
of a more obnoxious and harmful way to resolve differences. This guidelines seems almost certain to make
the physician-family relationship one of antagonism and
hatred rather than collaboration and compassion.
Dramatic threats to evict the baby can only destroy an
already fragile and complex situation.

Moreover, as Norman Fost notes, "More important,
if parents do yield to the pressure to take the child
home to die, the opportunity is reduced for persuading
them to change their minds, or to find other alternatives, such as foster care or adoption."[2] Threats of

this sort destroy a precious asset: time. Even if prepared, parents need time to adjust to the problem their
baby has, to sort out what is important to them, to think
about alternatives, to mourn for the baby they wanted
but don't have. The staff needs time to assess the
baby's condition, to perform tests, to evaluate how
different problems may interact with each other, to
evaluate what options are available, and to prepare a
plan of action. The baby needs time, too. Time to adjust to extra-uterine life, to respond to treatments, to
adjust to the environment of the newborn nursery. This
valuable time is lost if differences are resolved by dis-
charging the baby.

     Threats to discharge the baby to the parents may
coerce them to accepting a treatment for their baby that
they really don't want. We then have parents, already
alienated from the staff, coerced into assenting to a
procedure and having to care for a child whom they think
would be better off dead. Such threats have only profound negative consequences for all the parties involved,
especially the child.

     Another tragic outcome of coerced survival is the
hideously ironic situation of HHS's almost mandating that
all babies be kept alive regardless of their condition
while simultaneously the federal government, states,
cities, and private agencies as well are withdrawing the
financial support for facilities and staffing that provide the necessary extra-familial support to help such
infants survive and develop. Consequently parents who
are now forced to care for a child they feel may be
better off dead now have fewer social or financial resources to help them in this difficult situation. If
some people are afraid that denying treatment to infants
with birth defects constitutes child abuse, what will
they think about the social abandonment of these infants?

What is the long-term fate of a child with birth
defects who survives but is totally dependent on others -
the severely brain damaged but otherwise healthy child,
the child who requires frequent surgery, the chronically
ill child who has no hope of improvement, the child who
requires constant ventilation? Federal support for
individuals like this is rapidly vanishing and private
insurance companies can pay only so much. Will more
"accidents" occur at home? Will families be destroyed
to maintain physical life? Will taking home such a
child guarantee only unmitigated suffering?

Perhaps this act of discrimination - mandating
that a child live but denying support necessary to make
that life tolerable - is the act of discrimination that
needs the attention of the HHS. As it is, this second
guideline can only compound an already tragic situation.

So where do we go from here? What can parents do?
How can facilities and staffs respond? Because of the
complexity of the situation and the uniqueness of the
circumstances, no one set of guidelines will work for
everybody everywhere. Nonetheless, there are some steps
that can be taken to help clarify the situation and possibly alleviate some of the tension.

First, and I think this is one of the good points
implicit in the Directive, the facility should have a
clear, public policy on how children with birth defects
will be treated. Such a policy does not have to be framed
in "either-or" language, and probably can't be anyway.
But the policy should provide some clear guidelines about
what, in the light of the state of the art, realistic
alternatives are available. The policy might also suggest certain periods of review to ascertain what progress,
if any, has been made. what changes should be introduced,
the status of the infant, whether continued treatment is

indicated. This review can help keep individuals from
becoming locked into a situation and can legitimate
changing plans or trying different approaches. But in
any event, having an announced policy will help ensure
that all parties know where they are with respect to
the decision-making process.

Second, parents should be encouraged to seek some
counseling. A third party not directly involved in the
situation, while not disinterested or free of bias, can
more easily serve as a sounding board and provide the
opportunity for the parents to express their true feelings - feelings they may be ashamed of or think they
can't express to the nursery staff. Such counseling
will not make any decisions easier but may help clarify
different aspects of the situation, help the parents
acknowledge and come to terms with their feelings, and
provide a basis for decision-making.

Third, the parents should be provided with
information about the kinds of social services and
financial resources available in their community. This
will neither solve their baby's problems nor make any
decisions easier but again can provide a realistic context in which the parents can formulate a decision.
Knowing that they are not alone may help parents consider alternatives they would not otherwise entertain.

Fourth, parents must be kept up-to-date on the
condition of their baby. This is difficult because
the strain of the situation might keep some parents from
hearing what the staff tells them or because they deny
what is happening. Nonetheless, information is important because the medical condition of the baby is one
of the critical elements in decision-making. The staff
must be especially sensitive to the condition of the

parents. Information must neither be stuffed down the
parents' throats because "they need to know" nor presented so technically they can't understand. Rather the
staff must try to set a context which invites the parents into the nursery, encourages them to interact with
their baby, and helps them to learn what the baby's condition is, what is being done, and what is available.
Such gentle encouragement in this stressful time can help
the parents understand what is happening.

Fifth, the staff should encourage the parents to
ask questions. One way of doing this, as noted above,
is for the staff to take initiative in providing information. But another way is to reinforce parents' questions positively by answering them in a language that is
intelligible to them, not in medical terminology or with
a series of initials. The staff needs a professional
language, but they must also remember to translate for
the laity. Parents need to learn to say "I don't understand" or "would you please explain that again?" Again
the information provided may not solve any particular
problem, but it may suggest alternatives or limits on
the basis of which decisions can be formulated.

Sixth, all should recognize that the decision to
be made about the child's treatment is an ethical decision
or a value judgment. The test results, the data, the
diagnosis or the prognosis do not mandate any specific
course of action. What the staff and parents have are
sets of options, alternatives, and possible outcomes.
They have competent, professional judgments about possible
outcomes of various treatment alternatives. But knowing
what may or may not happen does not mandate a particular
treatment. What mandates treatment or denial of treatment is a value judgment about the worthwhileness of the
expected outcome. The medical data tells what is feasible,

not what must be done.   Our values, belief, and loyalties
tell us what to do.

I am not arguing that facts, data, a medical judgment are irrelevant or unnecessary. Our decisions must
be informed decisions, based on a realistic assessment
of options.   But in the final analysis, it is our assessment of the value of the outcome of these options that
is the decisive factor.   A child with severe brain damage
who is unresponsive may be kept alive through a respirator and other technical interventions.   But the fact that
a child may be so maintained does not justify doing it.
The tests and technical support systems tell what the
possibilities and limits of intervention may be.   The
physician's experience and clinical expertise indicate
what outcome may be possible.   Neither of these, however,
requires that any one option be followed.   That decision
is a value judgment.   The decision is formed, to be
sure, on the basis of expert opinion, but such a decision indicates an evaluation of the worthwhileness of one
specific outcome or treatment choice.   The facts of a case
do not mandate our decisions.   Our evaluation and judgment of what those facts lead to is what is ultimately
persuasive.

Thus far I have suggested several steps that can
help the parents, in conjunction and cooperation with
the physicians and staff, obtain a sense of what the
possibilities are and what course of action can be
followed.   The critical issue is on what basis should
value judgments be made?   What considerations are
most important?

One orientation, possibly standing behind the
HHS Directive, is that of respect for the sanctity of
life, or, to use the more popular, short-hand phrase,
a pro-life attitude.   This stance suggests that life is

the most significant value, that life must always be favored, that practices which threaten the fundamental value of life be prohibited. This orientation suggests strong intervention, using all available resources to preserve life. Life is preferable to death - regardless of the circumstances in which that life is to be lived.

This pro-life attitude is surely important and significant for our times. Proponents of this value have made us more aware of the forces of death and destruction in our society and more vitally aware of the disregard in which some lives are held. Such a pro-life attitude stands behind many powerful social movements which question war, capital punishment, defunding of social programs for the poor, and abortion. This pro-life attitude can be present in the newborn nursery and will evoke a strong preference to pursue whatever treatment alternatives are available. The goal is to maintain life, to affirm the life that manifests itself in the person of this newborn.

Another orientation, also very pro-life, argues that because life is precious and sacred we should pay careful attention to the circumstances in which it is lived. For these circumstances may so jeopardize life or require that all resources be devoted to the maintenance of life that living becomes impossible. This approach, focusing on the quality of life, presents itself in the newborn nursery by suggesting that the outcome of treatment be evaluated carefully. If the treatments do not offer some benefit or. which a realistic future may be based or if the resources available can only help to maintain the status quo, then the quality of life approach may suggest the denial or withdrawal of treatment.

Both of these attitudes are at opposite ends of a continuum - the continuum of life. If either is followed blindly or without being tempered by consideration of the other, serious harm may be done to the child.

If, for example, the pro-life orientation is uncritically coupled with the vast technical resources available in a modern newborn nursery, infants for whom there is no future other than a long, gradual, and complicated decline will be sustained by continual technical and medical interventions. This is done in the name of life but I would argue that life is served poorly if the best that can be achieved is a slow process of dying, accompanied by painful and stressful interventions.

The focus on the quality of life can also trivialize the life of the newborn by denying the value of the newborn nursery and rejecting those maneuvers that can demonstrably benefit the baby. Other values and preferences, masquerading as serious quality of life arguments, can put the child at risk of abandonment. Preference for one gender over another, a judgment about the career potential of the child - including athletic or musical capabilities - or estimates of the future economic burden of the child, can interfere with a serious evaluation of the child's potential and the options available to benefit the child.

How   parents use these orientations to judge what to do is difficult to predict. Probably they will not hold one extreme but will be more likely to bounce from one to the other, eventually settling on a direction which favors one part of the continuum.

One suggestion for helping both parents and staff to begin thinking through some of these problems is to attempt to separate decisions about treatment from both short and long-term care considerations. This can not be done totally, partly because responsibility for the care of the baby is a most critical aspect of the whole decision-making process and partly because we can't compartmentalize ourselves that easily. Nonetheless, this suggestion can help parents and staff to focus on the primary task: deciding what, if anything, can be done to benefit the child. Focusing primarily on that dimension of the process may cast some options in a clearer perspective. Separating treatment and care decisions may help parents and staff to reevaluate their priorities and value judgments.

Most importantly, perhaps, such a separation of decisions may help parents and staff to look at the interests of the child more carefully. If the parents can be helped to think about the child, his or her condition, the options and outcome rather than trying to work through long-term care responsibilities in a vacuum, then perhaps the best elements of the pro-life and quality of life perspective can unite to help parents determine the best interests of their child and what interventions or non-interventions may be in his or her best interest.

I recognize that this distinction between treatment and care decisions is artificial. But it may provide the parents with the breathing space they need to consider the medical possibilities and the interests of the child. Also, if the parents realize that they don't have to make all the decisions about the child simultaneously or within the first twenty-four hours of birth, they may be better able to put their energies to the most critical task of evaluating the possible interventions and their implication for the interests of their child. In this perspective, the value of life will be served but so will the interests of the child because the parents will attend to the circumstances which will affect the child's interests.

Making such decisions on behalf of a newborn will always be a difficult and tragic task for parents. Those who must make such decisions will be marked forever by them. To think of such decisions as anything less than tragic and painful would signal the ultimate devaluing of the life of the child and the indifference of the parents to their child.

Such a painful and difficult situation needs no more obstacles or burdens for the parents, staff, and child. Yet, this is precisely what I feel the Department of Health and Human Services is doing with its 18 May Directive. By seeming to mandate treatment without considerations of outcome or the interests of the child, the Directive places a far heavier burden than they need or perhaps can bear on parents, staff, and children. While well intentioned and understandable in light of the political atmosphere and the publicity given to some decisions regarding newborns, nonetheless such a Directive unfairly places a barrier between the facility, its staff, and the parents. Threats, fear, suspicion, lawsuits, and poor or coerced decisions are the likely outcome of this Directive if strictly enforced. The infant, the one whom the Directive is to benefit, can only lose by being placed in such a controversial situation. For the fate of the child and how he or she is treated will not be motivated by considerations of reverence for life or consideration of the quality of life, by the parents' love for the child, by their desire to benefit and do what is best for the child, but by motives of fear, threats of eviction, and labeling as bad parents.

Such attitudes can only work against the interests of the child and may prove to be a more significant handicap in determining what to do than the actual physical condition of the child.

FOOTNOTES

Norman Fost, M.D. "Putting Hospitals on Notice."
The Hastings Center Report 12 (August, 1982),
pp. 5-9. In this article Dr. Fost makes several
comments on this directive which I accept and uti-
lize in developing my own position and policy
recommendations. This article also contains the
full text of the HHS Directive.

Ibid., p. 7.

CULTS, MEDICINE, AND MENTAL HEALTH
Deviance and Difference

In the wake of the free speech movement, the anti-war movement, and the counter-culture movement of the late 1960's, a new current is appearing; a fascination with spirituality manifested by interest in eastern religions, mysticism, and the charismatic revival. Cultism is the blanket term for many of these new religious groupings based on alternate realities. Several of these groups have been singled out for special attention by the media, church groups, and concerned parents: the International Society of Krishna Consciousness, the Unification Church, the Church of Scientology, and most recently, the People's Temple, late of Jonestown. In addition to the questioning of their religious/theological foundations, there are allegations of brainwashing, mind control and the dehumanization of their members. Constant controversy surrounds the worship at these "alternate altars," as a recent book names these religious movements.

There are several thematic issues which are of considerable importance relative to the description and categorization of these religious movements. Although some problems are technical and sociological in character, they point to substantive issues which will shape how we think about these groups and their status within the community.

The use of the word "cult," poses the first problem. It is not too much of an exaggeration to say that the word has fairly pejorative connotations in both popular and most professional usage. Labeling an individual as a

member of a cult is a shorthand way of suggesting that
that individual is abnormal, deviant, and, in many instances, an ingrate. To describe a group as a cult, is
to label that group as critical of mainstream social
values, tyrannical, subversive, sinister, and enslaving.
In short, the word "cult" has acquired all sorts of nasty
connotations. Whether these are correct or not has
received little serious analysis.

The traditional description of a cult has been
within the church-sect categories initiated by Troeltsch
and Weber and developed by Niebuhr, Becker and Yinger.
Within this framework, the cult is seen as a privatiza-
tion of a dominant religion which appeals to the problems of individuals who are in some way deprived or disenfranchised. Membership in a cult also measures one's
distance form orthodoxy and is at its farthest extreme.
Thus, although cults are schismatic in origin, they are
still within the bailiwick of the church and, if viable
enough, may become established as a sect and eventually
evolve into a denomination. Within the traditional
framework, a cult is a way of testing individual or
group orthodoxy and social relations to the church. Although a cult stands at the extreme edge of orthodoxy,
it can provide a new explanation or interpretation of
the dominant religion, and, if successful, can become
an established sect or denomination.

Another description of a cult is provided by
Nelson.[1] In his view, cult formation is a way to analyze
the rise of new religions within a society and to measure
the growth of a dissident cult with a new vision into a
dominant, widely accepted belief system. In this perspective, cults arise from contact with alien cultures or
when the dominant culture can no longer provide answers
to personal and/or social problems, and, therefore, becomes

inadequate. Cults respond to this psychic and ethical
deprivation with their new vision which can give rise to
a new religion. If such a cult succeeds in becoming
institutionalized, a new religious interpretation of
reality occurs, and the old order passes away.

This understanding of cults - a test/measure of
social change/anomie - is particularly important for
current discussions of cults, especially those viewed as
destructive or religiously or socially deviant. First,
Nelson's view provides a more adequate account of the
tension - if not hostility - between members of cults and
other members of society. The cult provides the possibility of experiencing and expressing religious phenomena
in new modes and unconventional terms. This sets up
experiential barriers between the two groups. New values
and life styles emerge within the cult based on this
vision and are almost certain to be perceived as deviant
by the larger society. Traditional sacred authorities
will be challenged by the members of the cult because
they are responding to a new sacred authority. All of
these factors make communications between the two groups
difficult, if not impossible.

Second, if the cult is a response to the inadequacy
or decay of the traditional society, it will present a
direct threat to members of the larger society. Traditional visions of life, the deep and valid emotional
security that comes from sharing in an approved and workable understanding of life, and comfortable social roles
suddenly become vulnerable, especially if they are viewed
as optional instead of normative. We all resist change,
but resistance is highest when the foundation is challenged, and this is precisely what cults can do. Because
they strike at the culture's soft underbelly, cults are
viewed pejoratively.

Third, because of its new vision and the challenge it presents to the current order, a cult is devisive.
It can set child against family, friend against friend,
and newly born against the comfortably saved. Competition between new and old Gods has always been keen, but
this battle is particularly acute, for riding on the
victory is a new vision of reality, a new perception of
self, and a vision of a new social order. If it is true
that power is seldom surrendered without a struggle,
then this surrender will be all the more difficult because
it will be the Gods who do the surrendering.

The problem raised by Nelson's view of cults is
the traditional one of the old versus the new. The
question of the acceptability of values is of particular
importance here for both parties in the debate. Each -
the cult and the traditional society - view the values
and visions of the other with suspicion, alarm, and distrust. Differences in lifestyle and social relations
based on these values and visions are often incomprehen-
sible to the other. The new wonders why the old does
not see the beauty of the new experience; the old cannot
understand why these people think something is wrong
with traditional values. And because the old cannot or
does not understand the new, it must use the resources
available from within itself to answer its questions and
resolve its difficulties. Because the new typically
rejects the values of the tradition, it cannot appreciate
the significance of the old, and so the gap widens.

From a religious perspective, one can simply declare
the cultists to be heretical and dismiss them. Socially,
one can view the cults as yet another fad of the young -
a search for identity or self-assertion. If one is of
a more egalitarian or pluralistic mindset, then cults
can be seen as the pursuit of alternate lifestyles or

the living out of value options. Another more interesting approach is to view members of the cults as physically
and/or mentally ill. What makes this perception interesting and, possibly more dangerous, is that it uses the
traditional medical model to evaluate members of cults
and as the basis of intervention.

Establishing criteria to evaluate cults and their
members is extremely difficult, for one must be aware of
the uncritical acceptance of the superiority of one's
own values, unexamined claims of the normativeness of
traditional cultural institutions and mores, as well as
the limits of purely formal criteria. An example of
many of the problems one can face is provided by
Dr. Eli Shapiro, M.D., in an article entitled "Destructive Cults."[2] Although we find this article extremely
problematic and uncritical in its approach to establishing criteria, it provides an example of the pitfalls to
be avoided, as well as a demonstration of the tenuous
nature and limits of all criteria. After we present
Shapiro's orientation and our critique of it, we will
outline some perspectives on the evaluation of behavior
from religious and mental health points of view, and we
will conclude by making some comments on the place and
limits of criteria for evaluating behavior.

Shapiro's article focuses exclusively on destructive cults and their pejorative aspects; no mention
is made of what a constructive cult with positive aspects might be. Shapiro combines religious typologies
and the medical model as the basis for his critique.
Destructive cultism is described as a "sociopathic illness which is rapidly spreading throughout the U.S. and
the rest of the world in a form of a pandemic."[3]
Destructive cults are defined as those consisting of
characteristics which are harmful to the physical and

mental well-being of individuals and families. There is
a syndrome which includes personality change, loss of
personal identity, change in mannerisms, and psychological fear. Included in this menticide: "a dangerous
form of mental coercion in which the free mind is at-
tacked."[4] After an individual leaves a cult, either
voluntarily or following a process of kidnapping and de-
programming, medical management of this individual may
be necessary and can include a complete physical exam,
sedatives, as well as drug therapy, diet supervision,
hospitalization and psychotherapy.

The cults described as destructive have the
following characteristics:[5]

1.   Demands complete obedience to and
     subservience to one individual, who
     purports to be God, the Messiah, or
     some form of, or a messenger of the
     Diety.

2.   Requires separation from society.
     Association with non-members is
     discouraged except to gain money
     or to proselytize.

3.   Discourages any form of self-development.
     Education is scorned, and the self-image
     is totally destroyed.

4.   Teaches hatred of parents, organized
     religion and sometimes the U.S. govern-
     ment.

5.   Does not have concern for the material
     body; feels only the soul is important.

6. Takes all material possessions (past, present, and future) for its own use. Members are not permitted to own anything in their own names.

7. Makes it impossible for a member to leave, either through physical restraints or psychological fears.

8. Maintains the member in a "brainwashed" state through destructive behavior modification techniques.

These criteria do several interesting - and problematic - things. First, Shapiro claims they provide the basis for a diagnosis of an illness; yet, there is nothing of an explicit anatomical or psychiatric nature in the criteria. Second, the criteria are a means of identifying destructive cults, but there is neither an explicit definition of a cult nor a recognition of the different functions cults can play within a society. Third, the criteria assume, but do not justify, an image of religion and its relation to culture and social institutions. As such, Shapiro's criteria beg many questions and are easy to dismiss logically. Nonetheless, socially and practically, to many people they are appealing and comforting. And they do present a major dilemma: how to distinguish the deviant from the devout. Unfortunately, Shapiro answers this question without entering into the difficult and laborious process of argumentation and justification.

In this paper we wish to comment on problems in establishing and justifying criteria for distinguishing the devout from the deviant or the prophetic from the psychotic. In short, how can one critically address the substantive value issues inherent in determining the religious and mental status of a person, especially when that person presents a variety of nonconformist behaviors? Such a question becomes extremely critical when distraught parents bring a child or young adult to a physician or psychologist and demand to have this individual cured of his or her illness, the primary symptom of which is membership in a nontraditional religious movement.

In terms of religious evaluation, one's criteria, first of all, are related to and determined by where one stands. Thus, if one is a member of or a participant in a mainline, traditional religion, the tendency will be to view new religious movements through suspicious lenses because the movement represents schism or heresy. If one is a member of the new movement, one will tend to be led by its prophetic visions and view the tradition of the major religious denominations with condescension. Thus, each group will appeal to its own religious experience and/or doctrines as a means of condemning the other. And while one can perceive some of the possible personal and social implications of such experiences and doctrines, it is extremely difficult to evaluate these substantive issues without simultaneously making value judgements of one's own. This is where the traditional criterion suggested in the Christian scriptures - "by their fruits you shall know them" - breaks down, for it assumes a normative framework of categorization with valid criteria. This criterion also raises the problem of the authority/expert who applies it. It assumes that he or she has no interests or loyalties that could influence the judgement, that he or she is unaffected by values, or that this individual is in fact and actuality the ideal impartial observer. Finally, many of the implicit standards in such a criterion are subjective or based on intuition. This is not necessarily bad or wrong; it simply presents another area in which a variety of

values can emerge uncritically or unwittingly while
simultaneously maintaining a privileged position. Thus,
while this criterion presents an attractive standard, it
has within it a variety of problems that need to be over--
come before it can be used critically.

The Didache,[6] another ancient Christian document,
proposes a doctrinal and practical test. If the prophet
presents the teachings of Jesus and fosters righteous-
ness and knowledge of the Lord, the teaching is true.
However, if this prophet remains in a location for more
than three days, then that individual is a false prophet. Likewise, if a person requests money, he or she
is a false prophet. Finally, if the individual has the
behavior which the Lord would approve, then he or she
is a true prophet. Four criteria are proposed for discerning   such approved behavior: if the person orders
a table to be spread but does not eat from it; if the
person teaches the truth and does what he or she teaches;
if the prophet performs a mystery and teaches others how
to do it; if the prophet requests moneys for others
but not for self. True prophets and teachers are to be
taken care of and deserve food and drink; but those who
are false prophets and teachers, or those who refuse to
work, are to be turned out. They are "Christ-peddlers."
Such criteria rest on both commonly accepted values
and standards of a community and some subjective
interpretations of behavior. While some of the behavioral standards are more objective and less subject
to manipulation, the doctrinal standard admits of a
variety of interpretations and is less useful.

Jonathan Edwards, one of the foremost early
American Christian theologians, proposed a fairly extensive list of criteria in his work entitled Religious

Affections.[7] Edwards, of course, with his theological
presuppositions was in somewhat of a quandary. While he
wanted to be able to test the Spirit to discern the
godly from the ungodly, he was also aware that these
criteria could not be foolproof because of his religious presuppositions dealing with predestination and
the awareness of the certainty of salvation. Thus, Edwards very wisely deals with the affections, not salvation.
Genuine religious affections have their origin in spiritual,
supernatural, and divine roots. This source insures
that these affections will transcend natural or carnal
desire. They are based on the loveliness of the moral
excellency of divine things. These gracious affections
are also attended with what Edwards calls "evangelical
humility," the sense that a Christian has of his or her
own utter insufficiency and unworthiness. These affections also engender and promote a spirit of love,
quietness, forgiveness, and mercy such as appeared in
Jesus. Also, true religious affections are never satisfied in themselves, as false affections are: the higher
they are raised, the more the soul longs after a deeper
experience of these divine realities. Consequently,
these affections have their exercise and fruit in religious practice. That is, the Christian will live out
in the world the full meaning and reality of these affections, and thus they will be shared by all whom this
individual meets.

Operating out of the background of the psychology
of religion, William James[8] suggested three markers for
recognizing what he called theopathic behavior: purity
becomes twisted into a rejection/denial of both the
world and humanity; charity degenerated to a relation
between God and self to the exclusion of everyone else;
strength of soul precipitated into brittle self-sufficiency.

Even though these markers are rooted within orthodoxy and use it as a point of departure and a standard of comparison, they are not inherently tied to traditional social values. They help judge an individual's openness to reality and willingness to mature - which James assumes to be desirable.

From a different perspective, John E. Smith[9] points out three other criteria: the charismatic leader must point beyond self to an ultimate reality; the charismatic leader must be bound to the same standards and ethics as proposed for his or her followers; any money solicited must be put to visible human welfare and not reserved for the personal disposal of the leader. These formal criteria are reminiscent of the Didache, but deal with the major concern of many contemporary critics: personal integrity and fiscal responsibility. While fiscal responsibility can be reasonably easily documented, personal integrity remains a little more elusive.

All of these criteria point to very interesting dimensions of the practice of religion, but they all share in common a sense of rooting these criteria within an orthodox framework. Thus, what they are measuring is one's proximity to or distance from an orthodox tradition. The criteria are more accurately tests of whether one is schismatic or a heretic, or simply one who refuses to practice religion in a traditional and acceptable fashion. Armed with these criteria, members of mainstream religious traditions will always evaluate members of a cult unfavorably because the criteria are grounded in orthodoxy, not the possibility of allowing a new religious experience to come to fruition so it can be evaluated in terms of its own inner vision and strength.

Similar problems arise when one attempts to define mental health or to establish criteria by which one can determine whether an individual is mentally ill or not. One major problem is that mental health is often defined in terms of personality traits that appear to be highly valued by the analyst or the culture. Criteria such as these may tend to be less factual but no less normative than the physiological standards that one can find in clinical medicine. This orientation permits a variety of ideologies and values to become operative in an uncritical or unconscious fashion. For example, Karl Menninger[10] defined health as follows:

> Let us define mental health as the adjustment of human beings to the world and to each other with a maximum of effectiveness and happiness. Not just efficiency, or just contentment - or the grace of obeying the rules of the game cheerfully. It is all of these together. It is the ability to maintain an even temper, an alert intelligence, socially considered behavior, and a happy disposition. This, I think, is a healthy mind.

It would be interesting to determine how Menninger arrived at these particular criteria and values. Such a perspective leaves little room for questioning and challenging rules, even when it is apparent that they may need to be questioned. It also may be make it difficult to understand why an individual ought to experience righteous indignation; moral outrage is an appropriate response to some situations.

Another very clear indication of how values
influence perceptions of mental health is provided by
Mower's[11] summary of Alfred Adler's position on mental
health:

> A crucial consideration in determining
> normality is whether the individual is
> an asset or a burden to society and
> whether he is or is not contributing to
> the progressive development of man.

Such a perspective clearly relies on indications of social
worth and social contributions as key indicators of mental
health. It is unclear, for example, what the actual pro-
gressive development of humanity is. The claims of
General Electric to the contrary some forms of progress
may not be our most important or even necessary product.
It is also unclear how to evaluate the contributions
individuals make to society, especially when one tries
to compare short and long term gains. But the point is
clear - a definition such as this is based on values.

Another perspective on how values and defini-
tional issues influence each other is shown in Inge
Broverman's[12] research relating sex-role stereotyping
and clinical judgements of mental health. This study
hypothesized and demonstrated that clinical judgements
about "...the traits characterizing healthy, mature
individuals will differ as a function of the sex of
the person judged. Furthermore, these differences in
clinical judgement...parallel the sterotypic sex-role
differences previously reported." What Broverman showed
was that clinicians are less likely "...to attribute
traits which characterize healthy adults to women than
they are likely to attribute these traits to a healthy
man." A study such as this reveals clearly the significant role personal and social values and stereotypes

play in determining definitions or making clinical
judgements, both of which are traditionally viewed as
value-free. The conclusions show how the evaluation of
the behavior of others can be skewed because of the ideological basis of our criteria.

As difficult as the evaluation of behavior from
a religious perspective is, the issues become even more
complex from the psychological viewpoint. For when one
uses the religious criteria, at least there is a normative framework within which one can ground the criteria.
With definitions and perspectives of mental health such
as the ones quoted, we are forced to look for the grounding of the criteria in either the values of the analyst
or in the ideology of the culture. Both of these are
highly idiosyncratic and lead to certain definitions because of specific experiences and values. If one approaches individuals with definitions of mental health
such as these, it is quite easy to see that an evaluation of an individual who is acting differently will be
quite problematic and will pose a variety of issues that
need to be considered quite carefully.

For example, writers such as Fli Shapiro ask us
to accept the view that membership in a cult is, in and
of itself, symptomatic of the psychopathology of the
people who join and remain in it. However, in making such
a judgement, they do not adequately specify the criteria
which they employ to justify their conclusion. The
circularity of such reasoning is all too obvious. When
asked how we know that a particular individual is mentally
ill, we are told that he or she is a member of a cult.
To the question: Why is he or she a member of a cult,
we are told that he or she is mentally ill.

Shapiro and others are consistent in their approach with what has been, with one dramatic exception, a consistent theme in American psychiatry: the inclusion over the past few decades of an increasing number of behaviors within the category of "mental illness," demonstrated most succinctly by Zax and Cowan.[13] Contemporary psychopathologists also have as the object of their concern a broader spectrum of the population than their predecessors. But most importantly, the field of psychopathology is increasingly being defined by its study and treatment of people who do not define themselves as being patients. This distinguishes the field from the rest of clinical medicine. Just as alcoholics, drug addicts, certain criminals, and, most recently, cigarette smoking and shyness are listed in the American Psychiatric Association's Diagnostic and Statistical Manual of Mental Disorders, so too are we now asked to include a certain religious minority as, by definition, mentally ill.

It must be noted that while perceptions of what count as mental illness change over time, these changes frequently occur because the social climate and values of that particular time have changed, not necessarily because new knowledge has been obtained about a particular behavioral syndrome. Thus, even in the one exception to the historical theme of greater inclusivity of behaviors labeled as deviant - the decision by the American Psychiatric Association in 1974 to eliminate homosexuality from the category of sexual deviance - the decision resulted more from the social pressures of the gay community on psychiatry than it did from a gradual accumulation of scientific knowledge about homosexual behavior.

Psychiatrists and psychologists have never been able to arrive at a universally agreed upon definition of what constitutes either mental health or mental illness. The elimination of homosexuality from the list of psychiatric disorders was the product of a close vote among American psychiatrists, and there is still considerable debate and controversy in the field about the wisdom of that decision. The critical point is that in the absence of widely accepted standards of mental health or disease, it is incumbent upon anyone who labels a particular behavioral pattern as pathological in nature to specify the criteria being employed that justify that conclusion. Here, the argument represented by Shapiro is wanting - we are left with his opinion, an opinion which is inherently value laden but which fails to acknowledge the very existence of these values.

However, despite the lack of universal agreement about the nature of psychopathology, there is still enough agreement about mental illness that we are not reduced to the absurd position of having all behaviors be labeled as a disease due to pure subjective opinion or as a result of a majority vote of psychiatrists. One set of criteria for assessing behavior as psychopathological is proposed by Brendon Maher[14] in Principles of Psychopathology. The first is the subjective discomfort experienced by a person. When people seek psychological help to relieve the discomfort of emotions such as guilt, anxiety, or depression, they implicitly define themselves as deviating from other people or, more exactly, from what they believe other people feel. This subjective discomfort can exist even though the person's overt behavior is quite acceptable to themselves, and appears appropriate to the rest of the world.

Second, people seek help because of certain disabling behavioral characteristics or patterns which prevent more adaptive functioning in one or more situations. Examples are alcoholism, excessive passivity, impulsive outbursts of anger, etc. The presence of disabling behaviors may occur along with the person's being subjectively distressed about the behaviors, or may exist in the absence of any subjective distress. In this latter case, the person either agrees with, or goes along with, the opinion of someone else, usually a family member, that help be obtained for the unacceptable behavior.

The third criterion of deviance discussed by Maher is that of poor reality contact. This is the criterion most widely agreed upon by clinicians, even those of widely differing theoretical backgrounds, as indicative of severe psychopathology. An essential element of this criterion is the conviction that inherent to mental health and normality is accurate contact with and awareness of the external world. People who are not in such contact are readily labeled as deviant. Terms such as "psychotic," "schizophrenic," "delusional," etc. suggest that the person's reality testing is somehow impaired. As was the case with the criterion of disabling behavior tendencies, impaired reality contact may or may not be accompanied by personal distress. A person may believe that he is king of Jupiter and that static noises on the radio are communicating special messages to him, but he may not be bothered by these beliefs or define himself as needing help because of them.

Examining these criteria and attempting to integrate them into the argument exemplified by Shapiro and others leaves one with an almost impossible task. It cannot be argued that cult members automatically fit the criterion of deviance due to personal distress. Such a

criterion is, by definition, a self-imposed one. Just as
a person cannot be justifiably labeled as being unhappy
in a marriage or in a particular occupation if he or she
does not apply that label to him- or her-self, so, too, no one
could be described to be in subjective discomfort as a
result of cult membership, if the person does not so
classify him- or her-self.

When the second criterion of deviance is related
to the viewpoint of Shapiro, the situation becomes even
more confusing. Cult members can be classified as exhi-
biting disabling behavior characteristics in their voluntary actions if, and only if, one takes the position that
people should not spend their lives engaged in cult activities. Implied in this view is the idea that cult
membership somehow precludes a more adequate or better
response to life, such as active involvement in a more
socially approved religious organization would provide.
This view is neither correct nor incorrect in and of
itself; it is a value judgement and should be labeled as
such, although this is not done. The indiscriminate and
ideological use of the criterion of the presence of disabling behaviors helps justify the fact of cult membership as psychopathological in itself.

It is difficult to claim that membership in a cult
is indicative of poor reality contact. No mental health
clinician would agree to this in the absence of an intensive clinical assessment of each person who belongs to a
cult. Nor can it be claimed that cult membership is deviant because so few people in our society belong to one.
As Maher has pointed out, statistical infrequency of a
behavior is not justification for automatically labeling
it as pathological.[15] That is a lesson which should have
been learned when we think back only a few years and
realize the extent to which the early dissenters to American

involvement in the Vietnam War were labeled as socially deviant (and sometimes mentally ill) by American Society.

Another set of criteria for assessing behavior are proposed by Moor and Tucher in their analysis of delusions, a generally accepted sign of mental illness. They define a delusion as "a belief that a person has although he has (or at least has been presented with) considerable evidence against the belief, and comparatively little or no evidence for it."[16] On the basis of this definition, they consider a person to be delusional if and only if:

> 1. the person has a belief; 2. the person has (or at least has been presented with) considerable evidence against the belief, and comparatively little or no evidence for it; 3. the person has the ability to so evaluate this kind of evidence; 4. he would maintain the belief even if given ample opportunity and incentives to evaluate the evidence.[17]

What is immediately important about this orientation is that it avoids the problems associated with defining delusions as false beliefs (I believe my level of performance entitles me to a promotion) or deviant beliefs (Einstein's conviction of the correctness of the theory of relativity). That is, a person is not delusional because he or she misperceives a situation, has incorrect or inadequate information, or is among the first to have a new idea. Given appropriate evidence and the ability and desire to evaluate it, a person can correct his or her perceptions or develop evidence necessary to convince others of the correctness of his or her viewpoint.

The limitation of this orientation is that it is primarily oriented to individual beliefs and not the beliefs of a group. Beliefs about the ultimate nature of

reality, which form part of the belief structure of
religions, are difficult to test and because specific
evidence neither pro nor con can be gathered, Moor
describes these beliefs as unsubstantiated, not delusional.
The point here is that the theological structure of a
cult cannot necessarily be labeled as delusional because
of the beliefs of the cult. But if the beliefs of the
cult are not delusional, neither is the member who sub-
scribes to them - at least not on the basis of the beliefs. That is, a cult member may be delusional, but
not by virtue of accepting the beliefs of the cult.
The difficult problem here is to separate out those
personal beliefs which are delusional because there is
no evidence for them but evidence against them from
those framework beliefs which are unorthodox, different,
or deviant and have no externally certain evidence for
them or against them.

Nor does it follow that criteria which are appropriate for evaluating the psychopathology of an individual's behavior can be extrapolated to judge the "health"
of a social organization. One can describe the extent to
which a social system or a community contributes to or
detracts from the health of its members by observing the
effects of the system on its members, but that is a
very different process. We suggest that failure to see
this point leads to practices such as voting on whether
or not membership in a cult should be labeled as deviant
or devout, much as the American Psychiatric Association
did with homosexuality.

The critical issue is that the one doing the evaluating be clear on whether one is judging the religious beliefs or the personal beliefs of the individual. In the
former case, the more objective criteria for discerning
delusions can be appealed to; in the latter case, personal

value judgements can easily mix in with the objective criteria and personal beliefs can be uncritically labeled as delusional. Thus, within the viewpoint proposed by Shapiro, it is unclear how one can or, indeed, whether one ought to separate religious beliefs from personal ones or how one might understand and evaluate the interaction between them. Shapiro's framework is not helpful, therefore, because it collapses both framework beliefs and personal beliefs and provides no mechanism for identifying which is which or for evaluating either of them.

Throughout this paper we have mentioned different criteria used in distinguishing the deviant from the devout and have offered implicit and explicit critiques of these criteria. In light of that background, it would be less than fair of us to refrain from discussing how we view the evaluation process.

First, some preliminary comments are in order. One of our senses is that how one approaches this problem is a function of how libertarian one is. By this we do not intend to reduce the whole issue to one of tolerance, although that is important, but rather to indicate that that orientation shapes how one, first, sees certain issues and, second, how one structures one's response. For individuals who are concerned with order and the maintenance of traditional values, cults present a specific threat to society and the response must be direct and firm. For those who prefer difference and change, there is no threat and no issue. We feel that this fundamental way of seeing the world determines in large part whether one sees a problem or not, and, therefore, whether evaluation is necessary at all.

Another preliminary observation is that one can never be sure who the deviant are. In one instance it might be the Moonies or the Child of God or members of some Satanist group. At another moment they may be, as

is the case now, Hans Küng, Edward Schillebeeckx, or
Charles Curran. What this suggests to us is that what
may be important is not so much the criteria as the
authority which interprets and applies them. What is
critical here is how and what the authority perceives
to be occurring. We suggest that evaluational criteria
often take a second place to perceptions of threats to
the vested interests of the authority.

Another issue raised by attempts to evaluate cults
is the core problem of how, in our culture, to evaluate
the merits of rival value premises. That is, in a
pluralistic society, how does one discern the correctness or appropriateness of the premises upon which arguments are constructed? Because our society is built upon
the libertarian principle of individual freedom or non-
interference with individual actions, we have made it
difficult to define or accept a common value system.
Thus, while we champion individual rights and the civil
liberties of individuals, we are often reluctant to
evaluate what individuals propose to do with this liberty
of action. For example, it is obvious to most, if not
all, that the philosophy of the American Nazi Party is
wrong and deserving of condemnation. Yet in Illinois
and other places when the American Nazi Party has held
demonstrations, the problem was handled procedurely, not
substantively. Such a solution attempted to finesse the
value issue. However, the resulting debate in the American Civil Liberties Union suggested that the value issue
might be more important than the procedural one. So too
with cults; the focus of much of the debate has been on
ensuring the constitutional right of freedom of religion,
civil liberties, and due process. In the debate, the
real value issues have taken a back seat even though they
are really at the heart of the debate. Such a procedural

debate may be the appropriate focal point at this time to ensure that cults will be allowed to exist so that the real issue - the vision of reality affirmed by the cult - can be debated in another and more appropriate forum.

A final preliminary observation is that critiques of cults often miss features of them that are valuable for society. Deviant groups in general help define acceptable social and individual standards of behavior. Labeling a group as a cult, for example, points out what traditional society perceives as unacceptable religious behavior. It tells what, in the area of religion, is inappropriate. Such a negative evaluation has the positive effect of helping society become more self-conscious of its values, their implications, and their strengths and weaknesses. This provides the basis for an examination of these values with respect to their relevance for contemporary personal, social, and religious problems. From such a process can come a revitalization of traditional values and a new resolution of contemporary dilemmas. In this process, too, the values of the cult can become incorporated into the social framework and can make their own unique contributions. Second, a socially deviant group such as a cult gives disenfranchised or deprived individuals a place to go, a place where they can feel at home, or where they can receive some sense of usefulness or accomplishment. Such groups are helpful not only to those who are economically marginal and who are socially rejected, but especially for those who suffer ethical deprivation, the experience of value conflicts between the ideals of society and an individual or the experience of the inability to lead one's life according to one's own values and beliefs. A group such as a cult provides a place where these individuals can tell their story, pursue their values, and make contributions that are welcomed and appreciated.

The evaluational criteria we propose here are a combination of substantive and procedural norms. We feel this is appropriate because procedural criteria are rooted in our social framework and because substantive values are in part a function of interests and loyalties which need the moderation that comes from observing due process. Also, we are not totally sure ourselves of either what values we agree upon or which ones should be considered for widespread social acceptance.

First, we suggest that traditional religious or social values may not be the appropriate or only basis for evaluation of a cult. Precisely because a cult is typically based on a new or at least non-traditional value, it is neither fair nor just, at least prima facie, to judge or evaluate it by standards to which they do not subscribe or which might totally miss what they are about. One needs to determine: what are the values of the group; what needs, perceptions, or deprivations they answer: what appears to be the personal and social consequences of these values; do these consequences provide a resolution of needs that is satisfactory for the member of the cult? On the basis of these answers, the values of the cult can be known and this can form the basis for further dialogue.

Second, we could determine the source of these values. We do not intend for this to be a type of guilt or innocence by association or being judged by the company you keep. It is important to know whether something we perceive as different is different because it comes from and is an accepted part of a foreign culture or because it is a new revelation which an individual has received. Many of the groups people label as cults and judge pejoratively on the basis of the label are variants of traditions from Eastern religions. Even though one

may either misunderstand or disapprove of their values
and visions, at least a frame of reference is available
for understanding and evaluating them. Private revelations
do not always provide such a frame of reference and often
enough one is left with no good way to judge the revelation,
at least in the short run. Nonetheless, we know from
history that such revelations can be the source of social
movements that have significant consequences, for example,
the rise of almost all religious orders and the Protestant
reformation. From this perspective, it might be very
helpful to know whether social values or behaviors are
within the bounds of accepted cross-cultural variation.
While this will not necessarily testify to the worth of
the value, it might help us at least to be more tolerant
while we observe the behavioral consequences of the values
in question.

Third, autonomy and self-determination are extremely
important both culturally and ethically and if they are
to be respected and protected, individuals must be able
to choose and live out their values even if their value
choices are not the ones I or my society would approve.
We must insist that individuals are the ones who know
their best interests and which values are appropriate
for achieving them. To intervene in this process unjustly
is to limit liberty and to give one's own values a privileged position.

Fourth, as a consequence of the above, if we are
serious about engaging in the process of evaluation and
criticism, we must watch how the individual lives out his
or her values and listen to what he or she feels about
that experience. That is, one of the critical elements
in learning the worth of a value is understanding how that
value affects the individual who lives it. We think that
this is not a reflection of the philosophy of "if it feels

good, it is good" but rather is a recognition of the fact
that at least one part of a serious evaluation of a value
must be an observation of how the value functions and what
consequences it has. This cannot be hypothesized or based
on hunches - not at least if we are serious about evaluation.

We both share the sense that an individual's values
are very precious to that person and form, to a great
degree, the core of that individual's personality, as
well as provide the basis on which an individual can
evaluate his or her maturity and sense of integrity. We,
therefore, think that values should be interfered with as
little as possible, if at all. Because of our valuing of
autonomy and self-determination, we feel that individuals
should be allowed to choose their values and to devise
lifestyles that will actualize them. We suggest that such
values and their consequent lifestyles should be interfered with only when there is clear and substantive evidence of danger to a third party. This is a very traditional rule of our society, but one which we think serves
well in this situation. This procedural rule assumes
individuals have the right to determine their own lives
and to devise appropriate lifestyles but that when a third,
non-consenting party will be harmed by them, then an
individual's liberty of action may be limited. Please
note that we say limited, not completely removed. We
would argue that no one of us has the right to impose our
values on another individual although we might legitimately
limit his or her behavior. To safeguard this sense of
freedom and autonomy, we think that interference in the
life of another is justified only when there is clear,
substantive, and documented evidence of the possibility
of harm to a third party.

Another justification of interference would come
when an individual has or is suspected to have poor
reality contact. This would be defined by determining
if the person knows the answers to the traditional questions of who, where, and when. If a person shows by
correctly answering these questions that he or she is
in contact with reality, then we would suggest that a
wiser course of action would be to back off and leave
the person alone, at least until other evidence is
forthcoming. Of course, one problem with this orientation test occurs when the person seems to be out of
contact with what we would consider to be traditional
reality. But it does not seem clear to us that a
judgement of poor reality contact can be made necessarily when an individual claims to be in contact with
an alternative reality. That is, a person may claim
to have existed as different individuals in past civili-
zations, but still have good traditional reality contact. Thus, the issue may be deciding whether the
perception is a false belief or a delusion. Making the
judgement that such a person is out of contact with
reality can focus more on the reality dimension than on
the individual who is out of contact with it. Even when
using this fairly objective criterion of determining who,
where, and when, one needs to be cautious of uncritical
value assumptions slipping in and clouding the issue.

Our deepest sense from reviewing the cult literature and thinking about the issue of evaluation has led
us to the conclusion that evaluation is an extremely
problematic concept. When one suggests an evaluation of
a cult, one is already making an uncritical assumption of
the privileged position of one's own values or social
structure. Such a desire for evaluation also suggest the
irreformability of traditional values, as well as the

normativeness of the concept of tradition. What must be considered important in observing the desire for evaluation of cults is the very motivation for carrying out such an evaluation. We are not intending to escape the genuine problems involved in evaluations by such an attempt to turn the tables. On the other hand, we think it is very important to determine the motivation for an evaluation because we think that this will reveal a great deal about the values on which the evaluation will be made, as well as the adequacy of those values for such an evaluation. Therefore, if autonomy and self-determination are to be protected and enhanced, then society and its members must take the risk of allowing individuals to march to the beat of a different drummer or to see a vision re-vealed only to a few.[18]

FOOTNOTES

1. Geoffrey K. Nelson, "The Concept of Cult,"
   Sociological Review, 16:351 ff.

2. Eli Shapiro, N.D., "Destructive Cultism,"
   Association of Family Practice, 15:80 ff.

3. Ibid., p. 83.

4. Ibid., p. 81.

5. Ibid., p. 83.

6. Didache, 11:1-13:7.

7. Jonathan Edwards, Religious Affections. In The
   Works of Jonathan Edwards, Volume II, Ed. John E. Smith
   (New Haven: Yale University Press, 1959), p. 193 ff.

8. William James, The Varieties of Religious Experience
   (New York: Mentor Book, 1958, p. 256 ff.

9. John E. Smith, "Into the Secular Void," Commonweal
   16 mr, 1979, pp. 139-140.

10. Karl Menninger, The Human Mind (New York: Knopf, 1930).

11. O. H. Mower, "What is Normal Behavior?" In L.A.
    Pennington and Irwin A. Berg, eds. An Introduction
    to Clinical Psychology (New York: Ronald, 1948).

12. Inge Broverman et al., "Sex-Role Stereotypes and
    Clinical Judgements of Mental Health," Journal of
    Consulting and Clinical Psychology, 34:1 ff.

13. Melvin Zax and Emory Cowan, Abnormal Psychology
    (New York: Hold, Rinehart and Winston, Inc., 1972).

14. Brendan Maher, Principles of Psychopathology (New York:
    McGraw-Hill, 1966).

15. Ibid.

16. James H. Moor and Gary J. Tucker, "Delusions:
    Analysis and Criteria." Comprehensive Psychiatry.
    20 (July/August) 388 ff (1979).

17.   Ibid.

18.   David Finkel, Ph.D., a psychologist in the Depart-
       ment of Psychiatry at the University of Massachu-
       setts Medical Center, discussed several ideas in
       this paper with me and I am grateful for his help.

ETHICAL ISSUES
IN THE EVALUATION OF COMPETENCE

The purpose of this paper is to address three
problems: the social context of the relationship between physician and patient; models of competence and
their assumptions and implications; and an evaluation
of value issues that are inherent in the first two
problems.

The first section focuses on what I perceive to
be the shift in the physician-patient relationship from
an authoritarian one to a participatory one and the implications that this has for obtaining informed consent.
The second section of the paper focuses on the models
that people use for evaluating consent, but attends to
the value issues inherent in these in terms of the
assumptions that are made in using these models. The
final section highlights several problems thematically
addressed in the first two sections: autonomy, paternalism, and the physician-patient relationship.

I.   The social context of the physician-patient
     relationship

     A.   Changes in the Model of the Relationship
     In the traditional model of the physician-patient
relationship, which was clearly understood and sanctioned
by both physician and society, a patient went to a physi-

cian and described the problem; the physician listened to
what was said, took a history, made a diagnosis, and then
gave orders that the patient was to follow. The patient
then accepted these orders and at least occasionally did
what the physician said.

While such a description of the traditional relationship may be stereotypic, it nonetheless is reasonably
accurate. The physician played an active role; the
patient played a passive role. The role of the physician
was to give orders with the expectation that the patient
would follow them. The physician was perceived as having
the means, if not the power, to cure a particular disease.
The patient was perceived as powerless and not always
having the capacity either to understand what was happening to him or her or to evaluate it. In this traditional
model the only recourse that a patient had, if he or
she disagreed with the physician, was to change one's
physician. Challenging the authority of a physician was
simply not done.

A new social force has arisen within the last
three decades that has had a significant impact on this
traditional model of the physician-patient relationship.
I characterize this social movement generally as the
"rights" movement. In the late 1950's, our country
witnessed the development and approval of the Civil
Rights Movement in which blacks affirmed and demanded
their own civil and personal rights as citizens of the
United States. This movement quickly began to develop
in other areas so that in reasonably short order we had
the Women's Rights Movement, the Children's Rights Movement, Gay Rights Movement, Animal Rights Movement, and
Consumer Rights Movement.

On the one hand we can see the rights movement generally as an affirmation that people who are not members of professions or other powerful organizations are entitled to the same quality of respect and standards of justice and care that others are. On the other hand, the rights movement is a means by which various people who perceive themselves as disenfranchised have been able to gain some social and personal power and in this way to assert their own sense of personal worth and dignity. When one listens to the rhetoric of people in various rights organizations, one frequently hears a very aggressive tone of voice, occasional strident demands for the recognition and immediate implementation of one's rights, and strong claims that the one initiating the request is entitled to receive the service at least morally, if not legally.

The moral claims and rhetoric of this social movement are effecting a renegotiation of the physician-patient relationship. The issues center around power and control in which both parties in the relationship are perceived to be struggling either to maintain the power and control they had or to achieve a greater degree of these two qualities. Such a renegotiation of this relationship is extremely important in psychiatry because of the initial presumption that the patient not only is ill but also because in this unique situation the organ that is ill is the organ that we associate with consent to treatment. Thus a relationship that is already undergoing considerable social scrutiny is complicated by the quality of the perceptions that a particular patient may have both of the relationship itself and of his or her role within that relationship as it is articulated in terms of a variety of rights that patients are claiming.

B.   The Doctrine of Informed Consent

The doctrine of informed consent is, in my opinion, the basic ethical issue in all medicine. It is an ethical, cultural, and legal affirmation that people are entitled to approve of and consent to what others want to do to them before it is done, even if what is proposed to be done is in their best medical interest. The two important affirmations in this orientation are that people must know and understand what is proposed to be done to them and then they must give their consent to have this done. This orientation is based on traditional, ethical and cultural values such as freedom, self-determination, and autonomy. Taken together, these values affirm that individuals ought to be able to make their own decisions and that individuals are in charge of their own lives. This perspective suggests that in the medical context, the patient is the primary decision maker, is entitled to the knowledge that is necessary to make appropriate decisions, and must be free in determining what shall or shall not be done.

In general, informed consent is expected to contain the following items: (1) a full explanation of the procedures to be followed and their purposes, including identification of any procedures which may be experimental; (2) a description of any attendant discomforts and risks reasonably to be expected; (3) a description of any benefits reasonably to be expected; (4) a disclosure of any appropriate alternative procedures that might be advantageous for the subject; (5) an offer to answer any inquiries concerning the procedures.

As presently understood, the doctrine of informed consent affirms the obligation of providing information to the patient in proportion to what is needed by the patient to make a decision and to insure that the patient has an opportunity to consent or not consent to that treatment.

The moral and legal right to refuse treatment is a corollary of the doctrine of informed consent. The right to consent to treatment obviously implies the right to refuse treatment. There is a fairly lengthy case law tradition which upholds this right to refuse treatment which is based on the ethical values I articulated in discussing the basis for informed consent: freedom, self-determination, and autonomy. The claim is that if an individual is truly to be the master of his or her own fate and is truly to be autonomous, then that person must also have the capacity to act out those values which he or she perceives to be important. If one could not act upon these values, the right would be meaningless.

Affirmation of the person's right to accept or reject a particular form of treatment allows the individual to act out in society his or her values so that he or she may achieve the priorities that are perceived to be important and to incorporate them into a particular life style. This position defines the patient as the primary decision maker and claims that decisions about a treatment modality are primarily, but not exclusively, ethical or value decisions.

C. Implications

One of the clear implications of my previous discussion is that the physician-patient relationship is undergoing a significant amount of reevaluation. There is a definite tendency, at least in the literature, to describe this relationship no longer as a somewhat authoritarian relationship but rather as a participatory relationship in which each member has something to offer.

As this new model of a relationship is defined and practiced, a variety of problems will obviously arise. Both physicians and patients may be threatened: the former by a perception of a lack of power and control over the relationship; the later by the discomfort that can come from being asked to assume responsibility. Physicians may feel that their medical judgements are improperly being challenged by non-physicians. Patients, who now describe themselves often enough as consumers, may feel that they are not receiving appropriate levels of service and may respond accordingly. Many physicians may be very open to this model of a relationship and see it as a way of enhancing the quality of care they can provide for a particular patient but a patient may not wish to accept this responsibility and may continue to frustrate the physician in his or her attempts to make the relationship more participatory.

Even though the transition to a participatory model of the physician-patient relationship may be problematic, two important elements can occur. First, the physician can continue to exercise his or her traditional role as advisor of the patient and, in fact, this dimension of the physician's role could be enhanced. Second, values that are important to the patient and physician can more easily and quickly come to the surface and play their appropriate role in the relationship and treatment decisions.

A second implication is that many patients may make more demands upon physicians for information not only about the particular diagnosis and prognosis but also about the kinds of treatment modalities available and their life style implications. Thus a patient may request that a physician describe treatments other than his or her treatment of preference. Additionally, a patient may prefer a form of treatment with which a physician is extremely uncomfortable.

The new shift in an understanding of the physician-patient relationship and the emphasis on informed consent with its corollary of the refusal of treatment will continue to complicate the role of the physician with respect to the amount of information to be given, how that information is delivered to a patient, and dealing with how a patient handles that information, especially if the patient uses the information provided to refuse a particular treatment modality that the physician thinks is in the patient's best interest.

This social context in which decisions about patient care are made is extremely important and spills over into how competence is evaluated and especially in trying to understand some of the non-medical issues that stand behind assumptions of competence. This is especially true in psychiatry because there is frequently no anatomical base of reference for a diagnosis and because perceptions of diseases and symptoms are open to being influenced by personal or cultural values.

II.   Tests of Competence

The purpose of this section is not to argue for any one model of competence as normative. Rather I will present several tests of competence and their implications to clarify various ways in which competence can be perceived and to identify some value issues in determining competence.

I will describe five tests of competence and then discuss their assumptions.

A.   Tests for Competence[1]

1.   Presenting Evidence of a Choice.
This test is based on the observation that
a competent patient is one who can indicate some preference for or against treatment. The test does not evaluate the
quality of the decision but whether the
patient presents some kind of evidence of
a preference for or against treatment. This
test describes the incompetent patient as one
who cannot give any preference verbally or
behaviorally about a treatment modality.
If a patient does not protest a treatment
that is initiated one can infer, using
this test, that the patient is competent
and has consented.

2.   "Reasonable" Outcome of Choice.
This test focuses on the patient's ability
to reach what is perceived to be a reasonable
decision, that is, a decision that the physician thinks a reasonable person in roughly
similar situations would make. This test
does not focus on how the decision was
reached but on the fact that a person reached
a decision that is similar to one that the
physician thinks most reasonable people
would make.

3.   Choice Based on "Rational" Reasons.
This test for competency focuses on whether
the reasons that the patient gives for either
accepting or refusing treatment are rational,
that, is, on a determination of whether or not
they are a function of or a product of mental
illness. In this model, the quality of the

patient's reasoning process is critical,
not with respect to which decision is
reached, but with respect to how the reasoning process was used to arrive at the decision. This model defines the imcompetent
patient as the one whose reasoning process
is impaired by mental illness.

4.   The Ability to Understand
This model, quite close to the legal requirements for obtaining informed consent,
focuses on the patient's ability to understand the information that is presented
about the treatment. In this model the
patient's comprehension of the information
that the physician provides is more important than how the patient weighs that
information. This capacity for comprehension can be tested by the physician's
asking questions to determine the degree
and quality of comprehension. Once a
physician is satisfied that a person does
understand, that patient is then competent
to make a decision.

5.   Actual Understanding
In this model the competent patient is the
one who has actually provided a knowledgeable consent to treatment. The physician
must educate the patient and then ascertain
whether the patient has, in fact, understood.
If, in the opinion of the physician, the
patient has not understood, then the patient has not given adequate consent. This
model suggests that physicians must make
reasonable efforts to ascertain that their

patients understand what they are told and,
by implication, that they encourage active
participation in the treatment selection
process.

B.   Assumptions of These Tests

The first assumption of many of these tests of competency is a minimal ability to comprehend and evaluate
information provided by the physician. This further assumes some contact with reality, however minimal, and
some awareness of the consequences of either accepting
or rejecting the particular treatment strategy. Even
the minimal test of evidencing a choice is based on an
assumption that an individual can discriminate between
alternatives. This assumption leaves unstated the criteria by which one would test a person's comprehension
of treatment alternatives and also leaves open the more
problematic evaluation of a person's contact with reality.

A second assumption is that some reasons are more
reasonable than others. Such a situation is particularly
the case when a patient refuses treatment. My sense is
that in general there is a bias which favors the acceptance of standard or preferred treatments. This is
because the treatment has, in all likelihood, a high
probability of benefiting the patient and because a
physician or other health care provider has a strong
interest in providing services that he or she has been
trained to do and is skillful in doing. There is also
a social bias that if people are ill they should
receive treatment and resume their rightful position and
role in society. When a patient, then, refuses a treatment, such a refusal may fly in the face of a physician's
preferences as well as the social expectations of a person. The reasons a patient gives for refusing a treatment,
therefore, while convincing and meaningful to the patient,

may not be as significant or persuasive to other individuals.

A third assumption is the primacy of the rational
over other means of decision making. This assumption is
related to our society's infatuation with data, decision
making rules, and information processing systems which
give people at least the impression of control, if not
the reality. In this assumption the emphasis is on the
need to comprehend information, to relate this information to the situation at hand, and then to evaluate the
risks and benefits of the treatment in the light of the
information provided. Such an orientation is important,
but it is not the only one possible. Many, if not most,
of the decisions we make about ourselves have more to do
with our values, our conscious and unconscious motivations,
our fears and our fantasies than most of us are willing
to admit. Many treatment decisions may have more to do
with one's intuitions about mortality and immortality,
feeling about authority figures, or about the completion
of one's life project than a rational analysis of the
risks and benefits of a particular treatment strategy.
While an evaluation of treatment strategies from these
other perspectives are not inherently irrational, neither
are they as coldly rational as some commentators would
suggest is the norm for decision making.

A fourth assumption is that autonomy and self-
determination are the most important personal and social
values to be used as the basis for decision making. Such
an assumption assumes that each individual must make his
or her own decision, is responsible for his or her own
destiny, and, finally, stands by his or her own self because no one else can know what their best interests are.
I would argue that autonomy and self-determination are
important values and that at least prima facie they

should not be violated. On the other hand, I do not
think that such an assumption necessarily implies that
each individual is so isolated from everyone else that
his or her inner life is inaccessible. A narrow reading
of the value of autonomy suggests that each individual
is closed and inpenetrable by others; a more broad reading of autonomy would recognize the private core of
each individual but also affirm his or her significant
and necessary relations to society.

A final assumption is that most of the literature
that I am aware of focuses on competence as a static
concept and does not totally take into account the fact
that competency is a dynamic reality. To be fair it is
very difficult to develop an analytic concept of competency that is not static. One needs to sort of freeze
one's images so that one can analyze their component
parts. The danger and problem comes when commentators
forget that competency is a dynamic phenomenon and that
at different times individuals may exhibit different
degrees and levels of competency. This orientation can
be counteracted by recognizing that what one must do is
to engage in a process of evaluating competence, recognizing that having once declared a person competent or
incompetent does not resolve the ongoing problems that
a person presents in negotiating treatment strategies
with him or her. While viewing competency as a dynamic
concept presents many problems in that one must almost
continuously evaluate a person's mental status, such an
orientation is a more equitable resolution of treatment
decisions.

III.   Problems in the Evaluation of Competency

This section has as its purpose the analysis of
several issues to which I alluded. I would like to highlight several issues and talk about their implications
for competency.

A.   Autonomy.

As I mentioned a few moments ago, many commentators view the concept of autonomy as the major issue for
the evaluation of competence. In general, autonomy is a
form of personal liberty of action whereby the individual
determines his or her course of action in accordance with
a plan chosen by him or her self. The basic concept of
autonomy has two critical dimensions: 1) deliberating
on and choosing a course of action, and 2) acting upon
these deliberations. In this sense, autonomy is a
very traditional value in Western society and has a
special importance in the political ideology of the
United States. It is the ethical basis for arguing that
persons should be the masters of their own fate and that
individuals should be free to make decisions that are
significant for their own values and life style preferences. The value of autonomy helps ground the right
that we all assume that we each have to form our own
opinions and the right to be one's self. From this perspective, I think autonomy is in important value in
our own society. As long as we continue to perceive the
individual person as having dignity and as being a source
of values, I think we will also continue to value autonomy as the ethical value that helps the person articulate
the right to be his or her own self. However, as I suggested earlier, I think many people are assuming that

autonomy also separates one from one's fellows. Some
would suggest that each individual is so autonomous that
no one else can know anything about him or her or that
no one could possibly imagine what his or her interests
might be or how he or she might feel in a particular
situation. That is, my suspicion is that many people
are reading autonomy to be synonymous with a type of
radical individualism which removes the person from the
social context which we all need to grow and thrive as
human persons. This reading of autonomy would see
individuals as self-sufficent and independent of a social
framework which would help nourish their own development.

I think we should give a high priority to the
value of autonomy as I have defined it. On the other
hand, I think that we must recognize that to see a
person only as an individual is to short change that
person. To argue that a person must be left completely
to his or her own resources is to allow some individuals
to remain stunted in their own personal development or
to allow them to remain entrapped within circumstances
that they may not be able to control. The problem from
this perspective is trying to balance autonomy with the
recognition that a person at times may not be able to do
for him or herself what might be needed to be done. I
would argue for the legitimacy of attempts of society to
provide for people what they cannot provide for themselves, recognizing that one must begin such an argument
to provide these services with a high respect for the
individual's autonomy and his or her desires.

  B. Paternalism.

Very closely connected with the concept of autonomy
is its contrary, paternalism. In general, paternalism is
an intervention into the life of another person based on
the assumption that the one intervening knows what is best

for another person or what might be in his or her best
interest in a particular situation. Thus, paternalism
argues that another person's decision about what is in
his or her best interests should not necessarily be respected because of other considerations. Typically,
violations of autonomy are seen as paternalistic actions.

Ironically, however, often times a paternalistic
intervention can create a greater capacity for autonomy.
This is especially true in psychiatry and psychotherapy
in which the therapeutic process may enable the individual to define and then choose options which may not
have been available before therapy. The development of
various drugs has also been significant in terms of
helping restore a sense of personhood and autonomy to
individuals by relieving a variety of symptoms that
have interfered with people's decision-making abili-
ties. Thus, a paternalistic intervention has the
potential for opening up new life possibilities for a
person and enhancing their own sense of autonomy.

Again, while wishing to put myself on record as
being willing to recognize and justify paternalistic
interventions into the lives of other people to benefit
them, nonetheless I think we must recognize the tension
between the value perspective that a therapist, for
example, brings to a situation and the value perspective
of the patient. While I would be willing to argue that
it is quite correct to suggest that many people at
various stages of development do not know what is good
or best for them, I do think we continually need to
keep in mind that such interventions are primarily value
decisions and that it is easy to slip into a routine imposition of one's own values on another person, whether
this is done consciously or unconsciously. The problem
with paternalistic interventions is not completely with
the justification of the intervention but with the evalua-

tion and justification of the outcome with respect to a person's life project. Care must be taken at least to recognize the life project of another person and the value dimensions of that as well as the values of the therapist and society as one begins the process of justifying an intervention with that life project to help benefit the person.

C.   The Physician-Patient Relationship

I began this paper with an analysis of the changing situation of the relationship between the physician and the patient. I would like to conclude this section of the paper by talking about some dimensions of that that I think are important with respect to the discussion of competency.

A good example of the kind of issues that I am thinking of comes from the posthumously published article by Franz Inglefinger entitled "Arrogance" in the 25 December 1980 issue of the New England Journal of Medicine. Here Dr. Inglefinger discusses his reaction to the diagnosis of his adencarcinoma and the resulting quandary he faced when thinking through treatment options. Because his disease fell within his own area of specialization, he felt he could hardly think of a more informed and, therefore, competent patient. Yet he had trouble deciding whether he should receive chemotherapy, what kind of chemotherapy he should receive, and should he then receive radiation therapy. His own decision making process was complicated by the advice that he received from his family and from numerous physicians throughout the country. Relief came when someone suggested to him that what he needed was a doctor. Inglefinger concurred that what he needed was a doctor who would take charge of his case, be somewhat paternalistic, and would assume responsibility for decision making within the therapeutic

situation. Once this decision was made and a physician
selected, Inglefinger's quandaries and perplexity were
resolved.

   What this anecdote illustrates is the significant
qualities that a physician-patient relationship ought to
have as well as the kind of relationship it should be.
I would argue that a good way to characterize the kind
of relationship that should exist between the physician
and the patient is a fiduciary one. This kind of relationship is characterized by high levels of trust and
openness to the fairly clearly stated values of each
member of the relationship. In such a fiduciary relationship, both partners are respectful of the other's
values, although in this instance the patient more often
than not is willing to be led by the values of the
physician as they are articulated in treatment decisions.
In this type of a relationship, the physician focuses on
the good of the patient, assumes the role of advising
the patient, and accepts a high degree of responsibility
for the patient's best interests. This orientation does
not diminish the role of the patient nor ignore the
patient's values. Rather, the patient assumes that the
physician can see beyond the narrow interests of the
patient to what might be overall in the best interest of
the patient, from both a medical perspective, as well as
from the perspective of the person's life project. The
patient's autonomy and competence is complicated by the
physician's care and loyalty to the patient.

   In a fiduciary relationship, a physician will be
paternalistic and authoritarian, but not in a way to
demean the patient or to ignore his or her values. Such
a relationship allows the physician to have unique insights
into the patient and to have a sense of his or her interests as well as an understanding of the person's values

and what they mean to that person. Such information and insight is valuable in helping to ascertain the competency of the patient. And while this kind of a relationship is not always possible, it nonetheless provides a model for the kind of relationship that is most helpful in understanding the interests of a patient. Such an orientation helps the physician to avoid an uncritical paternalism and helps him or her to recognize the limits of autonomy that each of us experience. The fiduciary model of the physician-patient relationship allows the physician to go beyond a narrow contractual model and enter into a significant, personal relationship with the patient and to use the information that comes from this to help the patient articulate what is appropriate.

IV.   Conclusion.

Evaluating the competency of a person who is mentally ill is a complex and problematic task. In an age which focuses on individual rights and autonomy, such a task becomes even more complicated. I hope that my description of various models of competency and the assumptions that they contain will provide a framework that will be useful in analyzing one's own models of competence. Such an analysis will enable physicians to be both self critical with respect to their own value perspectives and socially critical with respect to cultural, political, and ethical issues that arise within the psychiatric context.

FOOTNOTE

1. "Tests of Competency to Consent to Treatment."
   Loren Roth, M.D., M.P.H., Alan Meisel, J.D.,
   and Charles W. Likz, Ph.D. American Journal of
   Psychiatry 134 (March 1977) 279-284.

ETHICAL ISSUES
IN THE USE OF COERCIVE THERAPIES

I.   Introduction

One of the most remarkable and significant phenomena
of the last decade has been the articulation and examination of ethical and value issues in the disciplines of
medicine, the life sciences, and behavioral sciences.
Of even more significance is the fact that many of these
concerns originated from practitioners of these disciplines.
Such concern reflects an awareness of the personal, social
and professional implications of research and practice
as well as a commitment to a high standard of professional
responsibility and commitment to the patient or public.

Such awareness is present in the disciplines of
psychiatry and psychology when there are many ethical
and value dilemmas, especially when treatment protocols
or strategies are planned and implemented. Such planning makes many value judgements about the patient/client
and his or her life style. Additionally, the patient may
be incompetent because of age, mental illness or mental
retardation and be unable to voice his or her interests
or values. When one of the treatment strategies includes
coercive therapies, the ethical complexities increase.

In the following sections, I will review policy
statements and proposed guidelines for dealing with
some of these issues, examine some thematic issues and,
propose a framework for an analysis of the ethical/value
issues in the use of coercive therapies.

II.   Review of Guidelines

    A.   American Association of Mental Deficiency

    In the April, 1975 issue of <u>Mental Retardation</u>
two sets of guidelines were promulgated which deal with
ethical and value dilemmas in the protection of human
rights and the use of various procedures in the treatment of mentally retarded persons. I would like to
indicate some salient features of these statements because I think they provide a good point of departure
and initial frame of reference.

        1.   Human Rights Review and Protection Boards[1]

    This policy statement defines a series of
mechanisms designed to protect mentally retarded persons'
rights which are susceptible to infringement because of the
economic, social, and personal situation of these individuals. This will be effected by establishing in each
state a board responsible for assuring the availability
of legal, administrative, and procedural safeguards for
these persons' rights. The boards are to review methods
and procedures for protecting rights, as well as any
legislation affecting these persons, serve as an independent review body, assure that service agencies have
due process appeals procedures, bring allegations of
rights' violations to appropriate agencies, and participate in on-sight inspection of programs. Such tasks
will serve to keep the issue of human rights before
administrators and the public. It will also serve as
a monitor, for even with the best of intentions and
programs, problems can arise but can be missed, ignored,
or hidden. The Boards will be of tremendous value in
addressing systemic problems in the treatment of the
mentally retarded.

2. The use of physical, psychopharmacolo-
gical procedures to affect behavior of
mentally retarded persons.[2]

The issues raised in these guidelines address
specifically the problems associated with devising and
applying a variety of therapies to modify a person's
behavior. The intent is to strike a balance between
providing potentially effective therapy and respecting the
vulnerability of the patient or subject. With respect
to individual plans, the guidelines propose the routine
and active participation of a client in selecting his or
her program goals and techniques, the review and periodic
assessment of the plan by appropriate review boards to
examine whether it is appropriate for the goals and whether
there is a minimal intervention strategy consistent with
reasonable and optimistic expectations of improvement,
rigid documentation of a plan which includes the updating
and changing of goals, the rationale for the selection of
strategies to achieve the goals and a documentation of
progress.

The guidelines also provide a review pro-
cedure which describes the problem of the setting of goals
and how they are to be examined. A distinction is
made between goals which are highly valued and generally
sanctioned by society (self-dressing, self-feeding, and
the elimination of behaviors which are harmful to the
person) and goals which are controversial (the elimination
of hallucinations or seizures, the development of certain patterns of sexual behavior and strategies which
weaken or strengthen certain types of assertive behaviors).
The review of strategies to achieve these latter goals
are to be reviewed on an individual basis and with respect
to the issues of: safety vs. danger to the client, the

enhancement vs. the dehumanization of the client, and the
demonstrated efficacy vs. the experimental nature of the
procedure. Also to be included in the use of controversial techniques are obtaining the consent of the client,
his or her participation in a selection of techniques,
specific review procedures, and a means of appeal. These
guidelines provide a frame of reference for classifying
therapies and criteria for the review of them which allows
both the reviewing body, the therapist, and the client
to identify and evaluate ethical/value issues to insure
and enhance the protection of the patient or client.

     B.   The National Commission for the Protection
         of Human Subjects of Biomedical and Be-
         havioral Research.

The Commission, which focused exclusively on issues
relating to research on human subjects, published reports
and recommendations which address the concerns of two
groups to which behavioral techniques might be applied:
children and those institutionalized as mentally infirm.
Even though not directly applicable to the topic of this
paper because of their being addressed to issues of
research, the Commission's reports nonetheless provide
an interesting perspective on some of the issues that
will be addressed throughout the rest of this paper.

        1.   Report and Recommendations: Research
           Involving Children.[3]

This report has two recommendations that are
relevant to our topic. Recommendation 4 states: Research
in which more than minimal risk to children is presented
by an intervention that holds out the prospect of direct
*benefit for the individual subjects: or by a monitoring
procedure required for the well-being of the subjects,
may be conducted or supported provided an institutional
review board has determined that: (A) such risk is

justified by the anticipated benefit to the subjects;
(B) the relation of anticipated benefit to such risk is
at least as favorable to the subjects as that presented
by available alternative approaches;...(D) adequate provisions are made for the assent of the children and
permission of their parents or guardians... Recommendation 7 of the Commission states: In addition to the
determinations required under the foregoing recommendations,
as applicable, the institutional review board should
determine that adequate provisions are made for:
(A) soliciting the assent of the children (when capable)
and the permission of their parents or guardians; and,
when appropriate, (B) monitoring the solicitation of
assent and permission, and involving at least one parent
or guardian in the conduct of the research. A child's
objection to participation in research should be binding
unless the intervention holds out a prospect of direct
benefit that is important to the health or well-being
of the child and is available only in the context of the
research.

There are several things of interest in these
two recommendations regarding children. First, the
Commission speaks of the child's assent, not consent.
By this the Commission indicates that a child is not
capable of giving his or her consent because the child
presumably cannot act autonomously. Rather, what the
Commission indicates is that the child should be asked
to determine whether he or she will agree to or disagree
with the proposal. Second, the Commission indicates that
a parent participate in the research by being present
during some or all of it. The purpose of this is to have
the parents sufficiently involved in the research so
they can understand its effects on the child and be able
to intervene if necessary. Third, the Commission
suggests that the parents' permission rather than consent

be obtained in order to distinguish what a person may do
autonomously from what one may do on behalf of another.
These elements in the recommendations help clarify the
relationship between the child and the parent with respect to the kind of things parents may do for children.
That is, parents may give their permission for a child
to engage in a certain kind of activity, but they cannot provide the child's consent. The other two issues
mentioned, the assent of the child and parental involvement in the research might also be transferable to the
therapeutic situation. By having the parents involved
in some way in the design and application of the therapy,
they can provide some assurance to the child that what
is being done for his or her welfare, as well as intervene on the child's behalf if that is necessary. Soliciting the assent of the child will incorporate the child
as much as possible in the research design and will give
the child an opportunity to exercise responsibility.
The use of the term "assent" does affirm, though, that
the child is not capable of giving consent and suggests
the continued monitoring of the procedure to determine
the child's reaction.

      2.   Report and Recommendations: Research
           Involving Those Institutionalized as
           Mentally Infirm.[4]

     In this report there is one rather lengthy
recommendation which is relevant to the discussion of
our topic. Recommendation 3 states: Research in which
more than minimal risk to subjects who are institutionalized
as mentally infirm is presented by an intervention that
holds out the prospect of direct benefit for the individual
subjects, or by a monitoring procedure required for the

well-being of the subjects, may be conducted or supported provided an institutional review board has determined that: (A) the conditions of Recommendation 1 are met; (B) such risk is justified by the anticipated benefit to the subjects; (C) the relation of such risk to anticipated benefit to the subjects is at least as favorable as that presented by alternative approaches; (D) adequate provisions are made to assure that no adult subject will participate in the research unless: (I) the subject consents to participation; (II) if the subject is incapable of consenting, the subject assents to participation (if there has been an ajudication of incompetency, the permission of a guardian may also be required by State Law); (III) if the subject is incapable of assenting, a guardian of the person gives permission (if a guardian of the person has not been appointed, such appointment should be requested at a court of competent jurisdiction) or the subject's participation is specifically authorized by a court of competent jurisdiction; or (IV) if the subject objects to participation, the intervention holding out the prospect of direct benefit for the subject is available only in the context of the research and the subject's participation is specifically authorized by a court of competent jurisdiction; and (E) adequate provisions are made to assure that no child will participate in the research unless: (I) the subject consents (if capable) and the subject's parent(s) or guardian give permission; or (II) if the subject objects to participation, the intervention holding out the prospect of direct benefit for the subject is available only in the context of the research and the subject's participation is specifically authorized by a court of competent jurisdiction.

Where appropriate, the institutional re-
view board should appoint a consent auditor to observe
the consent process and determine whether each subject
consents, or is incapable of consenting and assents, or
objects to participation, and whether the permission of
the guardian of an adult subject, or parent(s) of a
child, who objects should be supplemented by court
authorization.

Again, the Commission uses the distinction between
consenting and assenting to indicate the status of the
person's autonomy and the extent to which the patient or
subject can exercise personal responsibility. A second
significant dimension, which was also included in the
recommendation on children, is that the relationship of
risks to anticipated benefit must be at least as favorable
as that presented by alternative approaches. This provides an interesting context in which to review the risk-
benefit ratio, which is one of the major foundations for
the review of the ethical issues in research and practice.
While neither foolproof nor a guarantor of absolute
certitude, this rule of thumb can help devise a context
for evaluating the kinds of risks and benefits that a
person will face when he or she participates in a project.
This provides at least an initial way of evaluating that
ratio and incorporating it into a decision. Finally, the
subject's objection to participation can be overridden
only if the prospect of direct benefit for the subject is
available only in the research context and the subject's
participation is specifically authorized by a court. This
helps to insure a respect for the wishes of the subject
as well as a review of the procedure by an outside agency.

The issues that this recommendation deals with provide a framework by which we can think about some of the ethical dilemmas that arise in the application of a therapy to an individual. Of particular importance, is the recommendation that an individual's objection to participating in research that holds out the prospect of direct benefit can be overridden only by the availability of that benefit and by court authorization. What this might suggest is the necessity of independent review before a therapy is applied as well as taking seriously the objections the patient raises. Also by focusing on the fact that the patient can only assent to a procedure, the recommendation suggests a careful monitoring of the patient's continued participation and cooperation with a particular therapy.

III. Thematic Issues.

  A. The distinction between practice and research.

  In a recent article, Robert Levine[5] has clarified some of the terminological problems that have arisen over the past several years in discussions of the ethics of research and experimentation on human subjects. Levine analyzes how the National Commission used a variety of terms and proposed that we try to follow that usage. In general, practice refers to interventions that are designed solely to enhance the well-being of an individual patient or client and that have a reasonable expectation of success. On the other hand, research designates an activity designed to test a hypothesis, permit conclusions to be drawn and thereby to develop or contribute to generalize knowledge which will be expressed in theories, principles, or statements of relationships. These definitions set out fairly clearly the distinction between the two interventions but there is another intervention that seems to

be part of both. This is the class of procedures known
as nonvalidated practices. These are procedures designed
solely to enhance the well-being of an individual patient
or client but they may not have been tested sufficiently
often or well enough to meet the standard of having a
reasonable expectation of success. Nonvalidated practices are practices that physicians and other practitioners frequently use, but which have not been made
the subject of formal research. These practices benefit the patients but do not have the weight of research
behind them. Because of this, the Commission suggested
that nonvalidated practices ought to be made the object
of formal research to establish their safety and efficacy.

Such distinctions are important in applying
coercive therapies to patients. Many interventions
made on behalf of and for the benefit of a patient
emerge from different perspectives and orientations in
psychology and psychiatry and many of them fall into
the category of nonvalidated practices. And although
these practices do benefit the subject, it is important
at some point to do research to determine not only the
safety of the procedure but also its efficacy, so that
the therapist will know precisely what it is in the
intervention that is bringing about the beneficial
results. This would not only help the development of
psychology and psychiatry from a theoretical point of
view, but it would also be beneficial to the client in
that he or she would receive a much more carefully evaluated intervention. Such research would also address the
problem mentioned by Phillip Roos:

The possible effect of conditioning procedures
on the behavior modifier deserves special attention.
Procedures which lead to rapid and dramatic changes in
clients are likely to be highly reinforcing to the

behavior modifier and hence he is more likely to repeat such procedures. Care must be exercised, therefore, to ensure that the selection of procedures is not a function of the reinforcing effect on the behavior modifier.[6]

Addressing this problem through the development of well designed research protocols will promote both professional responsibility and concern for the client, and provide more appropriate interventions.

　　B. Issues concerning informed consent.

　　　1. Models of competency.

The problem of whether or not a person is competent to consent to treatment is an extremely important problem in almost every area of bioethics. It is extremely important and very difficult to resolve in the field of psychology and psychotherapy because the assumption is that the part of the person that plays a significant role in consenting - the person's mind - is the part of the person that is sick. While it does not necessarily follow that an individual who is mentally ill is incompetent to consent to treatment, many difficulties surround the means of ascertaining the person's competence. And even though minors by definition are legally incompetent to consent, there is the ongoing dilemma of what to do with the individual identified as a mature minor, that is, the minor who is older and more responsible for his or her behavior.

A variety of tests for ascertaining competency have been described.[7] The first test focuses on whether or not the patient can evidence a preference for or against treatment. This test is set at a low level and does not look at the quality of the patient's decision, but rather on whether or not the patient has affirmed or

rejected the proposed treatment. If there is no verbal
or behavioral preference expressed, the patient is considered incompetent. A second test attempts to evaluate
the patient's capacity to reach a reasonable or responsible decision. In this perspective, competent
behavior is what a reasonable person in similar circumstances would do. This test is, of course, biased in
favor of decisions to accept treatment and devalues
personal autonomy. A third test evaluates whether the
reasons for the patient's decisions are rational or
whether they are a product of mental illness. This test
focuses again on the quality of the patient's thinking
and is biased toward treating the patient even though
it is difficult to distinguish rational from irrational
reasons or to demonstrate that irrational thought processes in the patient have been because of the patient's
decision. A fourth test centers on the ability of the
patient to understand the risks, benefits, and alternatives to treatment. This test does not focus on the
quality of the patient's decision as the previous two
have, but on the patient's or client's ability to understand and process information about treatment. It is
really a test of the patient's ability to comprehend those
elements that are generally agreed to be necessary to
make an informed consent. This test focuses on how the
patient weighs and balances different elements, not on
how the patient evaluates this knowledge or the decision
that the patient reaches on the basis of the knowledge.
The final test argues that the competent patient is one
who has provided a knowledgeable consent to treatment.
The degree of competency desired and achieved is related
to the degree of sophistication that is desired by the
professional. Although more protective of the patient's
autonomy and values, such a level of competency may be
very difficult to achieve.

Although no one of these tests is probably used in its pure form, elements of all of them go into how we propose to test a patient for competence or evaluate how a patient has responded when we have sought to ascertain whether or not they will accept treatment. In each of these orientations towards competency there are a variety of subtle and unsubtle value issues to which all of us must attend. While we must determine whether or not the patient is competent, we must also be aware of what kind of values we are using as the basis of our determination of competence as well as how our own feelings about treatment refusal shape how we evaluate the status of the patient or client who refuses treatment.

2.   Problems.

a.   Age.

Age presents dilemmas of both ascertaining competency and obtaining consent at the two extremes of life: the very young and the very old. We know that the very young have neither the developmental skills nor the experience on which to base the decision of whether or not to accept treatment; we assume, rightly or wrongly, that many older persons have lost the ability to do this whether because of disease or the simple wear and tear of the aging process. A working assumption is that those in between these extremes, although perhaps occasionally impaired, have the competence to determine whether or not to accept a treatment.

One of the major issues that is important to think about when deciding whether or not to use a coercive therapy on a young person is their vulnerability, especially in terms of an inability to protect themselves from harm caused either by themselves or by other people, no matter how well intentioned or even appropriate their actions may be. Such a vulnerability, of course, becomes very critical when the behavior that the individual en-

gages in is self-destructive or extremely harmful to
him or her self.

Age also becomes a factor in devising
strategies of intervention because the older the child
becomes, the more capable he or she is of cooperating with
or resisting the therapy.   Thus, the issue involves soliciting the child's cooperation in therapy.   While it probably
is the case that a child cannot consent, we are safe and
correct in following the National Commissions recommendation that the child might be able, at some points, at
least to assent to the therapy.   Such attempts to involve the child in the therapy might provide the basis
of cooperation.   If such assent can be obtained one has
done as much as possible both to protect and enhance the
child's autonomy as well as to respect that child as a
person.   Oftentimes, of course, such assent cannot be
obtained and in these instances it is appropriate to use
the parents, guardians, or appropriate court officer to
provide permission to treat the child.   The important
issue is to articulate clearly how the proposed treatment is related to the best interests of the child.

b.   The need to treat.

As Roth and his colleagues note: "In
psychiatry the entire edifice of involuntary treatment is
erected on the supposed incompetency of some people to
voluntarily seek and consent to needed treatment."[8]   The
problem of providing treatment that appears to be necessary for those who either cannot or will not consent to
it is the source of many tensions and professional and
ethical dilemmas in psychology and psychiatry.   People
often engage in behaviors that are either destructive
to themselves or to other people or that are socially
inappropriate because they violate the mores of society.

It is often felt that such behavior is _prima_ _facie_ a
symptom of mental illness and provides the first level
of justification for involuntary treatment. Typically
the application of a coercive therapy or a therapy to
which a person does not consent is justified by one of
several means. (1) The freedom of an individual can
be limited when failure to do so will result in self-
destructive behavior.; (2) Individuals can be restricted
if their actions will harm innocent third parties.;
(3) The State can exercise its _parens_ _patriae_ power to
protect an individual when the State can demonstrate
that he or she cannot care for themselves.; (4) The
State can restrict actions that are offensive to the
sensibilities of members of the public. In each of
these instances there is the concern that what the
individual is doing will cause some degree of physical
or social harm to self or innocent third parties. The
intent of the treatment is to help the individual gain
the degree of control and autonomy that is necessary to
live as a responsible member of society. Problems arise
when necessary treatment is argued on the basis of lifestyle preferences relating to levels of assertive behavior, sexual activities, or the use of a variety of
mind altering substances, whether these be alcoholic or
pharmacological. Nonetheless, it is clear that some
individuals do engage in behavior that is physically
harmful and if left unattended could become self-
destructive. To leave a person in such a situation
would be to leave them in a situation almost worse than
one that could be devised by the most flagrant abuses
of psychology and psychiatry. In such instances intervention can be justified and the primary problems are
the effectiveness of the intervention and its appropriateness in terms of least amount of risks and fewest possible
side effects.

c.   Refusal of treatment.

The issue of the right to refuse treatment is one that has surfaced in the ethical, legal, and professional literature within the last decade. It is firmly established in both law and most of the literature of medical ethics that a competent adult has the right to refuse treatment. Such a refusal is premised neither on the quality of the person's reasons nor on their reasonableness. The fact that a person who is competent refuses treatment justifies the termination of any attempts to intervene in that person's behavior. Any intervention to treat a person after he or she has competently refused treatment would be legally an assault and battery and ethically a violation of that person's autonomy.

To hold that position, which I think is a correct position, is not to resolve any of the problems that relate to the refusal of treatment. It might be the case, for example, that an individual who is engaging in self-destructive behavior will not consent to be treated. An individual who is engaging in sexual activities that are not harmful, but primarily offensive, to other people will refuse to be treated for that particular problem. Two issues need to be evaluated. The first is the issue of public or private harm. The second is the competence of the person. I will refer to the previous discussion in terms of resolving some of the issues related to public and private harm. And although we have discussed issues of competency earlier, I think it is important to indicate once again that the fact that an individual is mentally ill does not imply that that individual is incompetent. Therefore we must engage in the tedious process of evaluating the patient's competence. We must keep in mind that when we wish to impose upon another person a therapy to which they have not consented or to confine them in an institution in which therapy can be provided, we are depriving that individual not only of his or her autonomy but we are also depriving that individual of his or her civil liberties. This is an extremely serious matter and it deserves our most serious attention and concern in evaluating the status of the person. The fact that an individual is a member of a profession and is skilled at applying therapies and is concerned about the health of other persons does not give that individual the right to impose a therapy on another person. The issue is not one of the ethical integrity of the therapist or his or her intentions. The issue is the competency of the person and whether he or she agrees to be treated.

Of course the issue will never be cleanly or easily resolved. It is important, I think, to approach the individual and to try to obtain either his or her consent or, if that is not possible, his or her assent to the proposed therapy. If neither of those are possible, and there is good evidence of harm to either self or others, then it is appropriate to approach the parent, next of kin, or legal guardian to obtain their permission to treat the patient. But the argument to treat patients against their will or without their consent must be carefully justified in terms of the interest of the patients and the harm that they are inflicting upon themselves and/or society. The goals of the therapy and the strategy to achieve those goals must be carefully defined in relationship to the values of the person and in terms of promoting the individual's autonomy. While such orientations will not resolve all of the issues attendant to this problem, they provide a beginning point which assures the appropriate respect for the patient as well as concern for his or her well-being.

        d.   The role of society.

        The values approved of by society often
play an unspoken but critical role in the evaluation of
the status of a person. While social conformity may not
have as high a place in the hierarchy of socially desired
behaviors that it formerly did, nonetheless society assumes that its basic values are correct and that when
an individual rejects them he or she may be manifesting
symptoms of at least deviance, if not of mental illness.
While the phenomenon of pluralism has been making steady
progress as the basis for arguing for the acceptance of
a variety of values and lifestyles that express them,
nonetheless the mores of society are important in
identifying individuals who might be ill and in justifying the kinds of interventions that might be sanctioned
to help such individuals recover. Attention to the
values of society is extremely important when the behavior in question is not or does not seem to be physically harmful to the self or others. This is not to
say that the behavior in question may not be disruptive
or problematic, but I think a line should be drawn fairly carefully between the two types of behaviors because
in the latter case the value issue is clearly present
and potentially problematic. Such problems usually focus
around sexual behavior, but they may also be related to
membership in religious cults, participation in demonstrations that are critical of governmental policies or
decisions, or rejection of sex role stereotypes. A
very profound issue that is raised by this question is
that of the loyalty of the therapist. Is his or her
primary loyalty to the patient, to the administration
of the institution, or to society? Is the therapist to
devise goals that reflect the patient's values or society's

values? Is he or she to help the patient to conform to the wishes of the administration or society, or is he or she to promote autonomy within the patient so that he or she can be free to make the appropriate decision? There will always be a tension between individual liberty and social order, and a therapist must be aware of his or her resolution of that issue and understand how that can affect a patient.

C.   Freedom.

Freedom is a highly desired and desirable personal and social value. When a person is free he or she is able to exercise autonomy and to implement his or her choice of values. Freedom provides a context in which an individual can exercise not only responsibility, but also self determination and can grow into maturity. Thus, it should always be with reluctance and sorrow that an individual's freedom is limited, even when it is apparent that this is being done in his or her best interests. This is why it is also painful and difficult to make decisions about treatments that are coercive, even though the ultimate aim of such a treatment is to promote the individual's freedom.

From one perspective, therapy is designed to promote freedom on the part of the individual and in the particular case of behavior modification it is to enhance the self control of the individual so that he or she might be able to exercise more autonomy. On the other hand, at least temporarily, the client is under the control of the therapist and the individual's behavior will not be free. Part of the therapeutic process is the deprivation of freedom in order to help the person control his or her self so that freedom can be restored. In therapy the person submits or is submitted to the control of another in the expectation that control by another will lead to control by self.

Such a deprivation of freedom, even though clearly arguable to be in the patient's best interests, must always be done with respect for due process and respect for the values and situation of the patient, in so far as this is possible. Thus I think it is appropriate to consider who it is who desires the behavior to be controlled and for what purposes. It is one thing to attempt to control the behavior of an individual engaged in self-destructive behavior such as head banging; it is another thing to seek to control the behavior of an individual because he or she does not conform to the schedule of an institution. Connected with this is an evaluation of who is exercising the control; the issue of interests and loyalties between the client, therapist, and relatives must be sorted out so that the best interests of the patient can be promoted. Finally, attention must be paid to the goals for the sake of which the individual's behavior is being controlled or modified. It is important to continue to focus, as a general goal, on the autonomy and freedom of the individual so that he or she can be in a better position not only to exercise the values of freedom and autonomy, but also so that he or she may more directly participate in the therapy and assume some responsibility for the process of being cured.

IV.   An Ethical Evaluation of Coercive Therapies:
       Some Considerations.
       A.   Thematic issues.

In setting out the framework for an evaluation of ethical issues in the use of coercive therapies, there are a number of issues that should be systematically brought to bear upon an evaluation of a particular therapy. While these issues do not specifically address each and every problem that will be encountered in devising and

evaluating a particular therapy, they provide a frame of
reference in which some major ethical issues can be identified and evaluated.

      1.   Respect for persons.

      The foundation upon which any evaluation should
be made is that of respect for the individual person or
concern for the dignity of the person. Attention to this
value will help ensure that all therapies are designed
to protect and promote the individual's autonomy and worth
as a person. It will help ensure that the person is seen
as an end and not as a means to an end. Respect for such
a value will also help the therapist and other members of
the team keep in mind that the primary reason for the
development and application of a particular therapy is
to allow the individual to attain a condition in which
he or she can make decisions by his or her self which
will implement the values that this individual feels are
appropriate for his or her life. If such concern is not
at the foundation of one's approach to therapy, it is
hard to understand how anything that is done for the
individual could be ethically valid.

      Concern for the individual and his or her
dignity would be of particular importance in evaluating
treatment alternatives that involve restrictions. While
recognizing that it may be necessary to restrict completely an individual's behavior, it should also be recognized that that is not necessarily the place at which
to begin a consideration of alternatives. Respect for
the individual would suggest that one begin with the
least restrictive alternative and then use other more
restrictive alternatives only when necessary. This
value would also help in the evaluation of the use of
noncontingent reinforcements as part of the therapy.

The kinds of noncontingent reinforcements selected should
be in harmony with perceptions of the dignity of the person as well as the use of means that will promote self-
respect and a feeling of personal privacy.

      2.   Goals.

      When setting out the goals for a particular
client or patient, it is important to evaluate whether
these goals reflect social, institutional, familial, or
personal values. While it is important to have the
patient/client be a functioning member of society, it is
quite possible that a variety of conflicts of interests
could occur between the patient/client and the therapist,
the institution in which the individual lives, or the
members of his or her family. Helping someone to become autonomous and self-determining is a risky business
for they may choose values or ways of acting that we find
reprehensible or outlandish. Yet one of the implications
of being free and autonomous is the ability to choose
behaviors that one wishes, whether these are socially
desirable or not. Thus, the therapeutic program may indeed help the individual to become autonomous and self-
determining, but may also facilitate that individual to
act in a way that is undesirable from the staff or
family point of view. This is where the question of
values that stand behind the goals of the therapy become extremely important in analyzing not only the goals
but also the conflicts of interests that might arise
between different individuals in planning out a treatment program and evaluating the results of that program.

      3.   The risk-benefit analysis

      For purposes of this discussion I will assume
that the benefit to be achieved by a therapeutic program
is either the removal of a particular behavior which is

harmful to the individual or a return of autonomy to
the individual. I am assuming that both of these benefits will be in the interests of the patient and will
help him or her to live an appropriate and meaningful
life in society.

However, even though these goals are extremely worthwhile, one must evaluate the strategies by
which they are achieved. One of the first issues to be
evaluated here is the efficacy of the program itself.
One must look at the program from the perspective of both
short term and long term gains to evaluate precisely how
the program will achieve the goals. One must also evaluate
the duration of the intervention. While time is not a
criterion to be used by itself, it is important to project
the expected duration of the therapy. This can have a
bearing on the acceptability of the therapy to the client
and the therapist, as well as help provide a framework
for evaluating the success or failure of the therapy.

The degree of coercion is another important
aspect to evaluate. Verbal coercion, even though not
physically invasive, can attack the psyche of the person in very profound ways   that can have significant
consequences. Thus verbal coercion should be evaluated
as carefully as, if not more carefully than, physical
coercion. Because of its potential for immediate as
well as enduring harm, physical coercion must be
evaluated extremely carefully. Whether the coercion
is external, such as the use of a shock, or internal,
through the use of a pharmacological agent, the therapist is exerting a profound control on the individual.
Thus specific attention must be paid to the kinds of
immediate harms that may result from the application of
this therapy. Care must also be taken to evaluate the

context in which the therapy will be used to provide
as great a degree of protection as possible. One should
also evaluate carefully the amount of pain that may be
attendant to the application of a therapy. This is a
tricky analysis because there is a clear intent to inflict a certain amount of pain or discomfort on the client.
The aim is to keep the amount of pain or discomfort inflicted at a therapeutic or tolerable level for the individual. Perhaps a rule of thumb might be that the amount
of pain or discomfort inflicted by a therapist could be
no greater than the amount of pain or discomfort the individual seems able to tolerate as manifested by the kinds
of behavior that he or she engages in. Such a rule of
thumb would point to an extreme limit of the amount of
pain that could be inflicted and one would assume that
one would increase the amount of discomfort only if there
seems to be no measurable benefit achieved by the level
initially selected.

      4.   Review.

      A final issue that needs to be stated is that
all treatment proposals should be reviewed by either an
institutional review board or the appropriate committee
for the protection of the patient at the institution.
The purpose of such a review will be to help ascertain
whether or not the client is capable of giving his or
her consent to the therapy or whether he or she should
be asked for assent. The review should also carefully
analyze the treatment proposal and its risk-benefit
ratio. The purpose of the review is to provide a wider
basis for evaluation than might be possible from one
to two persons who are closely involved with the patient.
A review board can serve as an excellent consultive
committee and can be of great help in promoting the
patients interests and developing a meaningful program
of therapy.

Two models for review.

A great deal of concern about these and other issues has been demonstrated by a variety of articles on the topic of ethical issues in the application and use of aversive therapies. Two articles provide an extremely interesting as well as comprehensive means of thinking through the ethical issues when devising and applying a program of therapy and I would like to present these as intra-professional ways of viewing the problem.

1.   Philip Roos: the minimizing of criticisms.[9]

Roos has devised a series of criteria which will help practitioners of behavior modification avoid a variety of both legitimate and illegitimate criticisms that have been leveled against it and also as a way of addressing the substantive ethical issues involved.   His criteria are as follows.

1.   Goals and objectives should be carefully selected to reflect the values of the client.

2.   Use of aversive consequences should be avoided or minimized.

a. Techniques relying on aversive conditioning should be used only when alternative pro-cedures have proven to be ineffective and/or when use of aversive techniques is advantageous over alternatives.

b. When aversive techniques are used, they need to be clearly defined and differentiated from procedures which are likely to meet with social condemnation.

c. Care must be exercised that the ends warrant the means.

d. The client or his advocate should be fully informed of the specific averse conditions which are to be used, and he should agree to their use before their initiation.

3.   Behavior modification should be systematically monitored on a continuing basis.

4.   Behavior modifiers should systematically involve key individuals and groups to insure maximum conformity with contemporary cultural values.

5.   Results should be continually subjected to scientific evaluation.

6.   Since the science of shaping behavior is in its infancy and changing rapidly, it is essential that the behavior modifier keeps current with research finding and new technology.

7.   Means must be carefully differentiated from ends.

These criteria provide a very excellent way of addressing many of the thematic and substantive issues that have been discussed in this paper.   Roos provides a way of promoting the respect for the person but also devising a therapeutic program that will be of benefit to that individual.

2.   Cook, Altman, and Haavik: a model consent form.[10]

These three individuals, who are involved in the use of behavioral therapies as part of their own professional work, have devised a model consent form which addresses many of the problems that they have encountered in obtaining consent or assent of clients. They include the following criteria as means to safeguard the rights of developmentally delayed persons.

1.   There should be a precise description of the aversive treatment procedure to be used.

2.   A description of treatment procedures that have already been implemented and their outcome is also necessary.

3. A description of treatment alternatives in addition to the proposed treatment procedure needs to be provided.

4. A justification of the purpose and rationale for the proposed treatment is needed.

5. There needs to be a description of any anticipated side effects or risks for the proposed treatment procedures.

6. Data recording procedures should be described and baseline data should be included.

7. The specific behavior(s) to be monitored need(s) to be clearly described.

8. The anticipated behavioral outcome including an expected time for the treatment to be effective should be described.

9. The qualifications of the persons who will be implementing the treatment procedures should be delineated.

10. The proposed treatment program should be reviewed by a Human Rights Committee.

11. Consent should be clearly informed based on the type of information presented above.

These criteria again reflect many of the details that need to be thought through in working out an appropriate treatment modality. While not as attentive to the social context as the criteria provided by Roos, these criteria are extremely helpful in working through many of the minutiae that are important in the designing of a treatment program that will be as respectful as possible of the rights of the individual.

FOOTNOTES

1.   "Human Rights Review and Protection Boards."
      an AAMD Policy Statement. Mental Retardation,
      April 1, 1975, pp. C-3-4.

2.   "Use of Physical, Psycho-pharmacological and
      Psychological Procedures to Affect Behavior of
      Mentally Retarded Persons." An AAMD Policy State-
      ment. Mental Retardation, April 1, 1975,
      pp. C-9-11.

3.   Report and Recommendations: Research Involving
      Children. National Commission for the Protection
      of Human Subjects of Biomedical and Behavioral. DHEW

4.   Report and Recommendations: Research Involving
      Those Institutionalized as Mentally Infirm.
      National Commission for the Protection of Human
      Subjects of Biomedical and Behavioral Research. DHEW

5.   Robert J. Levine, M.D. "Clarifying the Concepts of
      the National Commission." The Hastings Center Reports
      9 (June 1979) 21ff.

6.   Philip Roos. "Human Rights and Behavior Modifica-
      tion." Mental Retardation, June, 1974, p. 6.

7.   Loren Roth, Alan Meisel and Charles Lidz,
      "Tests of Competency to Consent to Treatment."
      American Journal of Psychiatry 123 (March 1977) 279ff.

8.   Ibid.

9.   Roos, op. cit.

10.   J. William Cook, Karl Altman, Sarah Haavik.
      "Consent for Aversive Treatment: A Model Form."
      Mental Retardation, February 1978, pp. 47ff.

HUNGER STRIKES

Blessed are They who Hunger for Justice

In the scheme of world events in which we are
accustomed to hearing of, reading about, or watching on
T.V. hundreds of thousands and even millions of people
dying in a variety of natural disasters or from the consequences of human intervention, it is somewhat ironic,
curious, or perhaps even bizarre that so much attention
is being paid to the deaths of ten men. It is even
more ironic, perhaps, because these deaths appear to
be freely chosen. They are not the result of a natural
catastrophe but are the consequence of an ideological
battle. Ireland has always captivated and even seduced
the attention of the world. She has done this in a
dramatic and forceful way with the IRA's decision to use
the hunger strikes once again.

The hunger strike has a fairly ancient history.[1]
It was known in the Far East as "fasting on one's enemy,"
derived from the practice of literally sitting upon the
doorstep of one's enemies either to humiliate the person
or to obtain revenge by inconveniently dying there. In
India the practice has a long tradition and has been used
by individuals to bring attention to their claims on
other people. In modern times the hunger strike was used
in Russia both by exiles and political prisoners under
the Czar to obtain some relief from their prison treatment.
There are records that as early as 1889, prison officials
responded to the hunger strike by forcefeeding women in
the Kara prison.

The hunger strike came to the attention of the world in the early 1900's as a consequence of the British suffragette movement. In 1909, a Ms. Dunlop was sentenced to one month in prison for printing on the wall of the House of Commons a clause from the Bill of Rights. To protest her imprisonment as a common criminal instead of a political prisoner, she engaged in a hunger strike. The prison officials were so caught off guard by this response that she was released after 91 hours. This caused the hunger strike to become an accepted, if not obligatory, weapon for suffragettes as they protested their status as ordinary or common criminals. Because of the popularity of the tactic and the continued resistance of the women to a variety of strategies to get them to eat, late in 1909, prison authorities adopted the tactic of forced feeding, typically done by inserting a tube into the mouth or nostrils and pouring milk and/or broth through it. Such processes invariably caused significant pain and resulted frequently enough in temporary and serious injuries. Many members of Parliament and physicians protested the use of this procedure but it continued to be used and the hunger strikes themselves continued. At one point there were several hundred women in British jails who were being force fed. This unwaivering fidelity to the discipline of the movement caused the Prisoner's Temporary Discharge for Ill Health Bill to be passed in 1913. This bill, nicknamed the "Cat and Mouse Act," permitted the authorities to release for a few days a hunger striker who was in danger of collapse. Having been released, she would then escape, only to be captured again and have the game continue once again. The impasse over the hunger strike with respect to the women's movement ended in 1918 with the passage of the Franchise Act which gave the women the vote.

By that time Irish Nationalists picked up the
tactic. It was first used by some Irish suffragettes
but was also used by a variety of nationalists in their
struggles for the freedom of Ireland. Two of the suffragettes were force fed for six weeks. In 1917, Thomas
Ashe, who was imprisoned for sedition, died as a result
of being force fed. His death led to the end of forced
feeding in Ireland but the British government continued to
resort to the Cat and Mouse Act. The effect of this,
of course, was to make imprisonment meaningless.

The hunger strike was also used by suffragettes
in America. One of the first to use it was Ethel Byrne,
Margaret Sanger's sister, in protesting her imprisonment of one month for operating a birth control clinic.
Prison officials, seeing that this tactic was being used
by many others, began a policy of force feeding. However,
there was a tremendous public outcry against the use of
forced feeding and it was abandoned. Many American uses
of the hunger strike by other members of the suffragette movement as well as conscientious objectors were
effective because of the policy of not force feeding in
America.

Ghandi used the hunger strike successfully
against Britain as part of his overall strategy for
achieving national liberation. In our country the hunger
strike was revived somewhat in both the Civil Rights Movement and also by the migrant workers. The use of strategies
such as the hunger strike and even more dramatic forms
of self-killing such as burning one's self to death as
was done by many individuals during the Vietnam War is a
way of indicating one's total commitment to a particular
cause, ideology or position.

People have always been willing to die for causes.
Why do the hunger strikers in Ireland attract so much

attention and how does one evaluate their position from
a moral point of view?

A.   General Background Information

Ideological clashes, of course, are nothing new
to Ireland. They have occurred since more than one person
inhabited the island. These clashes have been increasingly
more sharply drawn and more significant as the enemy has
become more clearly defined: the British, and especially
the British in Northern Ireland. One of the major problems
in evaluating and/or even understanding these ideological
clashes has to do with the fact that the Irish people
seldom seem to forget what has happened to them. While not
wanting to make superficial generalizations, it is the
case that the Irish seldom seem to forget their history,
their battles, and especially their losses. The losses
of a thousand years ago are still active in the Irish
mind and imagination. Events of centuries ago seem to
have occurred only yesterday and because of the continued
press of the reality of history upon the Irish mind and
experience, I think it is extremely difficult for those
in Ireland to achieve any degree of distance from their
past which would allow the possibility of some fresh
viewing of the relationship between Ireland and England.
Such a fresh viewing of the relationship may not improve
the situation at all; however it may be advantageous to
think of what might be done in the present as opposed to
using the present as a way of working out past relationships.

The use of the word "hunger" in hunger strike
generates many associations for the Irish. The most
obvious one is the great potato famine in the late 19th
century. The Irish, of course, do not call it a famine;
they refer to it as "the hunger." The potato was the only
vegetable that was struck by the blight. The usual grain

harvests occurred and the livestock was not affected by
the blight. These items, however, continued to be ex-
ported to England. The potato was the food of the peasant
and all else in Ireland was raised for England. Thus we
have the irony that during the 30 or 40 years of the
"hunger," there was plenty of food available but, nonetheless, at least three, and some estimate up to six
million, people died of either starvation or diseases
associated with severe malnutrition.

There were other options available and many
thousands of Irish emmigrated to the United States.
Many others remained and dealt with the reality of
Ireland. Seaweed became a very popular source of food.
Many Protestant churches opened up soup kitchens for the
relief of the starving Irish Catholics. Of course, the
Irish Catholic had a perverse way of dealing with the
Protestant soup kitchen. Those who took food from the
Protestant soup kitchens were perceived as traitors and
were labled as "soupers." They were expelled from the
community and normal relations with family and friends.
Even when times are difficult, one never collaborates
or gives the appearance of collaboration with the enemy.

One must also keep in mind the different distinct
but related dimensions of what is euphemistically referred
to as "the troubles" in Northern Ireland. The violent
conflict and revolutionary activities occurring between
the two sides seem, in some respects, to be the least of
all the problems. While one cannot contain terrorist
activities easily, at least one knows their sources and
their damage is typically finite, though it may be significant and intense. The more difficult problems relate
to the systemic problems in the society itself. Northern
Ireland is characterized by serious economic depression,
poor housing, incredible unemployment rates, and religious

and national hatred and bigotry that is being passed on
from generation to generation. In many respects the
most difficult part of the problem of Northern Ireland
has to do with the children who have been raised knowing
only conflict and violence and an atmosphere of severe
and significant hatred of the other side. All of these
elements combine to put an increasing amount of pressure
upon the different groups, either Protestant or Catholic
or Irish or British who are trying to seek political
solutions to the problem either through the political
process or terrorism and revolution. Underneath this
lies a whole way of life that is the first cousin to
terrorism: the routine stealing of cars and merchandise,
the continual harrassment of law enforcement officials,
including the army, and a general atmosphere of disrespect
for law and authority. Discipline is present but it is
most frequently meted out not by the law enforcement
officials but by the different terrorist groups keeping
order within their ranks. Knee cappings and beating are
the most popular way of keeping the troops in line. Knee
capping is also a particularly Irish institution. For it
guarantees the prolonged experience of pain and shame,
but without jeopardizing a person's life. It identifies
the individual as a problem person and helps segregate
that individual from the rest of society. Thus the
terrorist and revolutionary activities are in many
respects symptoms of the underlying problems of unemployment, disenfranchisement and poor housing. Whether
solving these economic problems would solve the political
problems of Ireland is unclear. What is becoming more
clear is that the terrorist and revolutionary activities
will not solve these problems either.

Finally, there are many issues involving the family and role behavior that are important to consider. One significant feature is that traditionally the most visible members of the IRA and its various factions are male and that all of the hunger strikers are male. In many ways this reflects the traditional role division in the Irish culture in which the woman remains at home and nourishes the family and the man leaves to engage in whatever activities he chooses, although several women went on hunger strikes in the early 1900's, including striking outside the entrance of the prison. Family life seems to remain intact even though there are tremendous pressures on the family from without and a sense of a growing lack of control over the family from within. It is amazing that any semblance of a normal family life can persevere throughout the several generations of conflict, but such seems to be the case and clearly the social structure of the family is viable enough to provide rudimentary socialization and the nurturing that is necessary to raise a family.

A critical point of tension with respect to families and the IRA has to do with the family watching its son slowly die as a result of going on a hunger strike. The moral tension is whether to respect the autonomy and decision of the son to participate in the fast or to break ranks and violate the discipline of the strike by having the son cared for. This typically happens after the striker become unconscious and can no longer control his own destiny, when the striker slips into coma and has only a week or two before death will occur. The pressures on the families at this time are especially great, particularly it seems for the mothers. In reported instances in which families have asked the striker to give up, the son reportedly will turn away or will ask that they leave. It is reported that Bobby Sands, the

first hunger striker to die, told his mother that if
she interfered with him after he lost consciousness and
if he survived that he would never speak to her again.
There have been, however, three recently reported incidents in which a striker's family has taken its son off
the strike after he lost consciousness. Two forces are
at work: the desire to respect the son's commitment to
his cause versus the desire of the family to keep the
son alive. There have been also reported incidents in
which families have encouraged their son to remain on
the strike after he gave an indication that he may
wish to leave it. One report alleges that a hunger
striker asked if he could have a glass of milk per day
in addition to the five pints of water and salt that
each of the strikers takes per day. He reasoned that
milk was a liquid and would not break his fast. Allegedly
one of the members of his family reminded the prisoner
that he had made a pledge to his commrads and then said,
"Remember, Bobby Sands is waiting for you in heaven."
The striker no longer asked for milk and died within a
week.[2]

    B.   Medical Issues

    Dying by starvation has always presented itself
as a particularly harrowing experience. The pictures of
the thousands of people starving to death in Biafra and
other third world countries as a result of famine, as
well as the pictures of individuals in different concen-
tration camps who have suffered extreme malnutrition have
always raised a tremendous amount of terror and anxiety,
as well as incredible amounts of appropriated sympathy in
observers. The terror of watching someone starve to death
is not lessened in the case of the hunger strikers because
they are doing it voluntarily. Now that ten strikers have
died, a pattern of the process of the strike and its se-
quellae has begun to emerge.

A great deal of special attention is given to the strikers by the other prisoners. They receive tremendous personal support from the prisoners. They are smuggled extra cigarettes, and special poems are written for them and recited within the cell blocks. However, after a striker has gone twenty-one days without food, he is moved into a hospital where he is placed in an individual room. Ironically this gesture confers upon him the status of a regular prisoner which is one of the goals of the hunger strike. Here the strikers are allowed to wear regular clothes and are allowed to have visitors. Radios and television are available to them and they will frequently hear special songs for them which are played by a sympathetic disc jockey. They are also allowed, again for the first time, to visit with each other in a room for two hours every evening. Each day they are weighed, and each day they refuse all medications and food and spend most of their time in bed as a means of preserving their strength. The strikers do accept sheepskin rugs in their beds to help keep them warm and they will accept a liniment rubdown from the nursing staff to soften their skin which begins to dry out. Almost like clockwork, on the forty-second day of the strike the strikers begin to experience nystagmus, a loss of muscular control due to severe vitamin deficiency. If the strikers look any direction but straight ahead, their eyes begin to gyrate wildly and uncontrollably. The disease also causes constant vomiting and nausea. The primary way to avoid many of the symptoms is to constantly stare straight ahead. Of course, this is almost impossible and the individual must go through the experience. The symptoms typically end after about four days and the relief from its terrors provides the strikers with a period of both physical and psychological relief.

However, as the strikers get deeper into the
strike, other symptoms begin to occur such as the slur-
ring of speech, the failing of the senses of hearing,
sight, and smell. The strikers then slip into a coma
and eventually quietly slip into death.

This pattern is known to the strikers and even
though they may not be able to appreciate all of the
things they will experience, especially the symptoms of
nystagmus, they go into it knowingly and being aware that
more likely than not they will die. Hourly reports are
broadcast within the prison to the other prisoners and
everybody is quite aware of what happens, when it happens
and what the ultimate fate of the strikers will be.
However the men in the prison are tough and the strikers
seem to be the toughest of the tough. In many ways they
exemplify the words of a hunger striker who died in
1920, Terence MacSwiney, the Lord Mayor of Cork, who
went for seventy-four days before he died. He said:
"It is not those who can inflict the most, but those who
can suffer the most who will conquer." The arena in which
that premise is being tested is the bodies of the hunger
strikers.

The Central Ethical Committee of the British
Medical Association made a statement on hunger strikes
in 1974. [3] One may have trouble finding the statement
because it is not indexed under hunger strikes but rather
under the heading of The Artificial Feeding of Prisoners.
That is a quaint euphemism to describe the process of
force feeding an individual. It is also an interesting
way to define what the problem is.

The immediate context of this statement's being
drawn up seems to be the force feeding of at least two
sisters in a British prison from 3 December 1973 until
the end of their strike on 18 May 1974, as well as the

death of a IRA member after a 60 day fast during which he
was intermittently fed artificially. Michael Gaughan
was in jail because of his participation in a bank rob-
bery but went on the hunger strike to be reclassified
as a political prisoner and returned to Ireland. The
medical officer who attended Gaughan in prison said that
there was no question of his being mentally ill and that
he felt bound to respect his patient's wishes when he
declined treatment and consequently Gaughan was fed only
when he became seriously weakened. The cat and mouse
game of the previous century seems to be in progress
here also.

The statement of the Code of Ethics with respect
to the forced feeding of prisoners is an attempt to
respond to problems like these. There are two basic
ethical principles being argued throughout this statement. The first of these is the common perception that
a medical officer would be negligent of his or her duty
if he or she let the health of a prisoner on a hunger
strike be endangered without attempting to help.
When it is necessary to consider forced feeding, the
statement says,

> "In this procedure a prison medical
> officer must be given complete clinical
> independence in deciding for or against
> the course of action under consideration.
> The priority between an obligation to pre-
> serve life and an acquiescence with the
> the prisoner's wishes is one which doctors
> may assess differently, with equal sin-
> cerity, and the decision must take account
> of the prisoner's physical and mental
> state as well as the wishes which he may
> have expressed on the subject."[4]

The question the statement deals with is whether
a physician ought to stand by and do nothing in the
case of what could be described as an attempted suicide,
even though the patient has not consented to the treatment. The decision to intervene and force feed a prisoner
is based on statements drawn from the Declaration of
Geneva and the International Code of Medical Ethics. Both
of these codes argue that a physician must have the ut-
most respect for human life and that a physician must
attempt to preserve human life and not use medical knowledge in a way that is contrary to the laws of humanity.

The other ethical principle that the statement
uses is that of freedom of clinical judgement on all
matters involving patient care. The statement argues
that in the case of prisoners who refuse food and do not
show any signs of serious physical or mental illness, as
long as they are age 16 or over and of sufficiently sound
mind to understand fully the consequences of their decision to withhold consent and cooperation, a physician
may choose not to intervene and that physician will not
be regarded as guilty of any professional misconduct.

One of the other sub-themes in the statement on
the artificial feeding of prisoners has to do with the
allegation that such forced feeding is unethical and
constitutes a form of torture. The two responses that
the statement makes to this are: 1) a physician is
obligated to respect human life and act to preserve
human life; 2) a distinction should be drawn between the
consequences of a voluntary act by a prisoner who has
been properly tried and sentenced in this country and deliberate physical or mental torture by a totalitarian
authority with the object of obtaining information from
subjects who have not been tried in court.

One can infer from the tone of this statement that it does not perceive force feeding to be a form of torture. Also the statement begs the question of a proper trial since a person may be arrested and detained for up to a week without being charged with a crime, although there is the requirement of the person's having some association with terrorist activities.

The hunger strike presents many medical-ethical problems, especially with respect to issues of force feeding a patient, the continued palliative care of individuals who continue on such fasts, and general concern about the appropriate role of the medical staff in these situations. Issues relating to appropriate exercises of paternalism become important as well as how do health care professionals implement and act responsibly with respect to both their professional code of ethics and their own personal consciences.

C. Ethical Issues

The first issues concern problems related to autonomy, paternalism and coercion. In general, autonomy pertains to a person's capacity both to choose a plan of action and then to have the capacity or ability to implement that plan. Autonomy is an important value because it is the way that we achieve self-determination and manifest control over our own lives.

Paternalism, on the other hand, is some intervention into the life of another person either because that person is incompetent to decide on behalf of his or her own self or because we think that, even though the person is competent to decide on their own behalf, that person is making a decision which is not in his or her own

best interest. Thus paternalism is a way in which individuals or society show concern for the lives of other
people by attempting to protect them when there is a
danger of harm or when they are incapable of choosing
for themselves.

There is, of course, a significant tension between
autonomy and paternalism. One individual may see the
decisions of another as extremely harmful to that person
but the actor may perceive that these actions, even though
containing a high risk of danger, will eventually prove
extremely beneficial and in fact are extremely desired.

Coercion refers to a person's being forced to do
something other than what he or she may wish whether this
be by another person or by the environment in which one
lives. There are a variety of subtle and unsubtle ways
by which we can be coerced or perhaps even seduced into
doing those things which we do not want to do. Advertising
is perhaps the most blatant example of seduction of the
autonomous agent. Peer pressure and membership in various
social groupings also exert various forms of coercion
on us.

Coercion is an important consideration in the
hunger strikes insofar as it is at least legitimate to
ask whether or not the individuals would volunteer if
they were not in the particular situation in which
they are. Many individuals argue that prisons in and
of themselves are terribly coercive environments and
that they diminish a person's autonomy and consequently
weaken their will to resist. It is also important to
consider whether membership in the IRA or the Irish
National Liberation Army exerts a degree of coercion over
the members so that they are really not sufficiently
distanced from their situation to consider adequately
the consequences of what they're doing. Family membership

is also important with respect to both trying to stop a
person from going on a strike and to encourage a person
to keep going with the strike. It is almost impossible to
obtain any perspective on what is actually happening in
the prison so that one can evaluate the degree of coercion.
It's clear though, that the IRA is a fairly tightly defined group, has its own internal code of honor and code
of discipline and that they are totally committed people.
It's also the case that the IRA receives enough support
to make it a viable organization and it continues to be
attractive enough and to provide enough of an alternative
to draw new members. It's also the case that, contrary
to what many people expected, the problem is not obtaining enough volunteers for the strikes but rather trying
to choose from among the hundred or so that have volun-
teered which ones will be the next to stand in line.

Paternalism is also an important issue with respect to the strikers both from the point of view of the
jailers and from the point of view of the families. It
seems reasonably clear that the IRA will not actively
intervene to attempt either to change a person's mind
about going on a strike or to argue that they should go
off the strike once they have started. The British,
for the most part, have adopted a hands off policy
and are letting the strikers play out their hand to
the end. Some parents are beginning to intervene and
override their son's decision to die by having him fed
after he slips into a coma and can no longer control
his own destiny. There are several reasonably good
arguments for making paternalistic intervention which
could be employed, in fact are relevent to this particular situation.

Generally speaking, to justify a paternalistic
intervention in another person's life one needs to:
1) demonstrate that there is a serious risk of harm to
a person who is incompetent; 2) the harm to be prevented
or the benefit to be provided outweighs the loss of
independence or the other benefits that the patient seeks
in taking his or her actions; 3) the paternalistic intervention should have a reasonable chance to prevent the
harm; 4) it should be the last resort and the least restrictive and insulting means of intervention should be
employed. Of course, that is a formal or procedural
argument and serious questions have to be raised with
respect to the value system on which one's argument would
be based for weighing risks or for evaluating the benefits the actors hopes to obtain. Clearly an intervention into the life of a hunger striker will stop the
striker from dying and in that sense will stop a significant harm from occurring. However, preventing that
harm may in fact stop the benefit that the striker wishes.
Thus even though one can construct a reasonably good
procedural argument one continually needs to attend to
the value issues that stand behind such an intervention.[5]

A second issue has to do with the problem of
labeling or how we identify people who have taken specific strong stands. Another way to articulate this is to
think through the basis on which we identify and locate
the hunger striker on the scale of intensity or totality
of commitment to a particular cause. We have in our
history any number of individuals who at least open themselves to the possibility of dying, if they do not directly place themselves in a situation in which death is
a likely outcome. We are familiar with the martyr, the
soldier, the patriot, the spy, a civil rights demonstra-
tor, the Budhist monks and other Americans who burned

themselves to protest the Vietnam War; we know, from both
the tradition but also from the television series, of
the Jews at Masada who killed themselves rather than submit to Rome, we are reminded frequently of the people at
Jonestown, some of whom were probably murdered but some
of whom may have committed suicide; we are continually
confronted with patients who submit to very risky procedures because such a procedure may be their only possibility of survival, we have people like Evel Knievel
and other stunt drivers who expose themselves to high
levels of danger, we have individuals who volunteer to
be subjects in medical experimentation and research
which exposes them to high levels of risk. We can come
up with a rather lengthy list of individuals who, for
a variety of reasons, are willing to expose themselves
to high degrees of danger and risk of danger or even
to the likelihood of dying.

What is interesting in making such a list is
trying to determine why some of these individuals are
highly valued by society for what they do and why other
individuals are denigrated or have aspersions cast upon
their character because of what they do, even though the
consequences may be the same for both groups. Thus, for
example, we expect a certain degree of heroism in our
soldiers, dramatically illustrated by the fact that we
expect some soldiers to be the first to land on the
beach of an enemy, even though it's quite clear that
most of those will be killed. We have all been provided
in elementary school with the inspirational figure of
Nathan Hale who regreted that he had but one life to
give for his country. Many people marveled at the
courage blacks exhibited during the civil rights demonstrations when they exposed themselves to extremely high
levels of physical and personal danger both to demonstrate

the totality of their commitment as well as the immorality
of the segregation laws. When we think about something
like Jonestown or even Masada, however, a completely
different set of feelings might be evoked that are primarily negative. Many people would assume that such
deaths were useless and perhaps even stupid and were done
without any good reason whatsoever. This may also be
the case with our evaluation of those individuals who
burned themselves to death to protest the conduct of
the United States during Vietnam. We may also feel this
way about the comedian Dick Gregory who also underwent his
own fast, drinking only water, to learn what the effects
of starvation are upon the body. The hunger strikers present another example to use in thinking about the kinds
of issues that are raised when we observe behavior that
is at one end of a spectrum.

The problem here, of course, is how do we identify
behavior that is at the end of a spectrum. Is it fana-
ticism, is it extremism, is it simply a person's commitment acted out to its full consequences? Important in
this, of course, is the kind of value perspectives that
we pull in consciously or unconsciously to evaluate the
particular action.

This particular issue raises a third problem which
is related to how we begin to identify and evaluate these
types of ultimate commitments. Whenever we see someone
willing to go all the way with their commitment, we are
forced to raise the question of, to what ought one totally
give one's loyalty or, to phrase the question in the way
Paul Tillich, a prominent Protestant theologian did,
about what or whom should one be ultimately concerned?
How does one evaluate where people put their faith,
their loyalty, their trust? Typically people have given
this kind of loyalty and concern to their nation, to

various political causes, to various ideals, to various
organizations, or to one's God. Often enough such personal commitments do not cause problems with respect to
the evaluation of the actor's behavior. But on the other
hand, we know that such basic beliefs are now beginning
to show up more and more frequently in a variety of
political contexts and, as a result, have increasingly
a public dimension. And people are being forced,
whether they like it or not, to take some sort of a
position with respect to evaluating these behaviors.
Once people begin to put their beliefs into action, it
becomes increasingly difficult to avoid evaluating the
behavior because of the necessity to make some sort of
a response to a social change. The issue then becomes
how does one's personal ideology whether philosophical,
religious, or political influence one's perceptions?
All of us see from a particular vantage point and we
need to be conscious, especially when we are arguing
that our vantage point is professional and not ideological, that nonetheless there is an influence in our
perception by our ideology. Thus one person's martyr
may be another person's fanatic. One of the major
problems that we have in our particular pluralistic
society is that we do not have a set of common premises
anymore by which we might socially evaluate the actions
of different people. That is, I think that it is the
case that consensus is becoming something more and
more difficult to achieve because each of us, to varying degrees, is going more and more in his or her own direction
and consequently losing contact with other people. In
many ways we are seeing played out in this country the
logical consequences of a liberal society and of a
rather complete acceptance of the value of autonomy or
self-determination. While this is an important value,
one also needs to think about what the consequences of

radical autonomy are for the social system. I suggest
that one problem has to do with the difficulty in achieving a
sense of consensus or coherence within the society so
that we can as a culture evaluate different problems.

A fourth issue relates to the problem of what I
will call self-killing. I am using the term "self-
killing" rather than suicide because suicide typically
has pejorative connotations associated with it and for
the purposes of a moral analysis I would like to try to
keep those pejorative feelings somewhat at a distance.
What I would like to do here is talk about some of the
traditional ways of analyzing the morality of self-
killing and trying to provide some examples as a way of
entering into thinking about the morality of the actions
of the hunger strikers.

Let me provide a few ways of thinking about self-
killing. The traditional distinction is between self-
killing that is indirect and self-killing that is direct.
In an act of indirect self-killing, one's death was not
desired or aimed at but rather was a consequence whether
foreseen or not of an otherwise legitimate action that
one would wish to perform. Such an indirect self-killing
was perceived in the main by the tradition as justified.
There are many examples of this. The most typical is
that of a soldier throwing his body on a grenade to save
his friends. Another typical example is that of the
martyr who dies rather than violate the integrity of his
faith or betray his faith. One could also think of a
person who would give his or her place on a lifeboat to
another individual. In direct self-killing, the intent
is to cause one's own death as something that is desired
for its own sake or as a means to an end. Here death is
directly intended as the primary consequence of the action.
Typical actions that are prohibited as unjustified acts

of direct self-killing would be to kill oneself because of a psychological depression, because one is out-of-control or because one is suffering and one wishes to end the pain.

There are several basic arguments which are used to support the moral prohibition on direct self-killing. These include: 1) the taking of one's own life is contrary to our own natural instinct to love life and to conserve and preserve it; 2) self-killing is an offense against society, for by taking one's life, one deprives the community of a good; 3) life is a gift of God to humans but only God has direct dominion over life and death and therefore killing oneself oversteps the boundaries built into the structure of reality; 4) an individual may be incompetent and therefore may not be able to decide for him or herself.

There have also been a variety of arguments developed to justify indirect self-killing: 1) the public good may be preferable to an individual good. For example, a physician may expose him or herself to the risk of incurring a fatal disease during an epidemic so that he or she can care for other individuals; 2) helping a neighbor in spiritual need may be a greater good than preserving one's own life. The typical example up here is a chaplain ministering to soldiers in battle, exposing himself to the risk of death in order to provide spiritual consolation to those who are dying; 3) the good to be done may outweigh the possibility of one's own dying. The typical example here is the one mentioned previously of a person yielding his or her place in a lifeboat to someone else; 4) a good for one's self might justify exposing oneself to some risk of death. One is entitled to take the risk of a dangerous operation for the benefits that it may bring.

Both of these frameworks provide again structural or procedural ways that we can use to think through whether an act of self-killing may be justified or not. I think, in summary, that the common moral tradition argues that killing is not good and because of that self-killing is also not good. However, there is room in this to overcome the presumption of killing's not being a good so that individuals are morally entitled to engage in various activities in which there is a risk of death or exposure to a significant degree of danger of serious harm for other compensating goods. The different kinds of self-killing that I have alluded to provide interesting test cases both historically and contemporaneously which stretch this teaching to the limit.

Martyrdom, for example, has traditionally been one of the accepted forms of self-killing. Yet it is the case that many of the Christian martyrs appeared quite anxious for martyrdom. It is reported that Saint Ignatius of Antioch requested that when it was his turn to go to the arena that people should not try to hold back the lions because he was so eager to be eaten by them. There are also reports that many of the Christian martyrs would eagerly throw themselves upon the fires that were prepared for them so that they could more quickly achieve the crown of glory that awaited them for their fidelity. There are also reports of many Christian women who preferred death rather than have their virtue violated by the pagans.

Other moral dilemmas are presented to us by our contemporary world. For example, it is reported to be a common practice for highly placed espionage agents to carry with them a cyanide pill to use to kill themselves lest they reveal important information and/or the identities of other agents under torture. Torture is also being used as a routine means of interrogation in many countries and questions are raised about the morality of individuals killing themselves before they are tortured so they do not either reveal correct information or make false statements about other people because of the severity of the torture. These situations are quite common especially in third world countries where there may be active guerilla warfare occurring but also where there may be radical, revolutionary, or democratic political movements. The moral proposal here is that self-killing is justified when there is a probability of breaking under torture and harming other individuals or jeopardizing the success of a movement.

This leads into a discussion of the moral tension between self-killing that is justifiable and that which is not. To a large part the morality of self-killing hangs on the perception of whether the self-killing has the quality of sacrifice to it. That is, those forms of self-killing with which individuals feel more or less comfortable and which in fact the moral tradition sanctions have to do with those actions which are perceived as having a noble aim. Self-killing is justified when it appears to be for the benefit of another person or when one's act of refusal to save one's life appears to be to promote some good, whether this be social, political, or religious. Self-killing, therefore, appears to be most justifiable when the act involves some type of other regarding motivation. Those acts of self-killing which appear to be selfish or which have as their intent the removal of the self from some problematic reality, appear not to be as justifiable or in fact are not justified by the moral tradition.

It is in the light of these different elements
that one can begin to approach some of the moral issues
with respect to the hunger strikers. Part of the moral
evaluation depends on the different ideological issues
involved; the legitimacy of defining the IRA prisoners
as political prisoners as opposed to common, although
important, criminals; the legitimacy and significance
of the question of a united Ireland; the perception of
the suppression of what would be a Protestant minority
if the North were to be united to the Republic of Ireland.
Our evaluation also would depend upon what people think
are appropriate limits to nationalism and patriotism.
It would also depend upon one's basic perception of
the legitimacy of the cause of the IRA. And, how one
perceives these different issues will also be influenced
by how closely one may want to stick to technical and/or
professional definitions of delusions, obsessions, or
mental disorders.

In many ways the hunger strike is the limit case
for the morality of self-killing. From one point of
view, the hunger striker neither wants to nor intends
to die. The expectation is that the gesture of refusing
food will reveal to the other party the seriousness of
one's cause, the depth of one's commitment, and the
willingness to be totally committed to a course of
action. The assumption is that such a demonstration will
persuade the other person to change his position or at
least to begin negotiating some compromise. As a factual
matter, however, it appears that the British Government
is going to be as equally intransigent in its position
as the IRA is in its. Therefore, one can expect that
those who go on the strike know that they will die.

One can argue that the ideological, political, and social beliefs of the hunger strikers are both sincere and strong enough to allow the definition of their actions to be categorized as instances of justified self-killing because they are sufficiently other regarding in character. The hunger strikers are not committing an act of self-killing which is a function of depression, or which is a signal of their being out of control in a way which might justify typically some intervention. On the basis of the scanty evidence available the hunger strikers are quite knowledgeable in what they are doing and are doing it so that they can achieve their political goals. The issue of whether this is an appropriate strategy is a separable issue and even though individuals might perceive the strategy as misguided, the wisdom of the strategy may not undercut the morality of the gesture itself. Enough analogies can be made with soldiers, those fighting in revolutionary movements, and even those involved in guerilla warfare to make one think that going on a hunger strike is also a justifiable form of self-killing because one does not seek death in and of itself and because one is trying to achieve goals that are of benefit to other individuals.

There are two other issues with respect to the hunger strikers that I think are important to bring out. The first has to do with the issue of control of one's life in an extremely confined situation such as a prison. A hunger strike may be a way in which a prisoner is attempting to achieve some control over his own life and destiny in a situation in which he does not have that control. This point is made in one of the few references to hunger strikes in the professional literature. While it is important to remember that these comments are made in the immediate context of the Soviet prison system, it is also fair to recognize that there have been many documented cases of torture of the Irish prisoners in the Maze prison. The following quotation is instructive in that it provides some psychological orientation to what is occurring.

> "This recourse to a particular form of non-verbal protest may be the result of differences in personality, degrees of self-consciousness and emotional capacity. Political prisoners are mainly non-conformists. Unlike the ordinary criminal recidivists, they are oriented to people and social issues and their imprisonment derives from a concern with moral principles and ideals. The functionaries of the Soviet prison system often consist of unscrupulous persons who themselves seem to have strong criminal and psychopathic inclinations. Political prisoners are treated very roughly and cruelly. Wardens wish first of all to establish a moral victory over the political prisoners by forcing them to do something dishonest, for example, they try to make them denounce their friends and fellow prisoners. In this way, they attempt to place them within the social category of the criminal.
>
> Despite the impossibility of asserting their rights of physical freedom, political prisoners always try to win a psychological victory by achieving 'internal freedom' and independence. Because of this, they choose the passive mode of protest, characteristically a hunger strike, a device by which the prisoner asserts control over his own fate and his own body.

Therefore, both the hunger strikers and those
who mutilate themselves in other ways remove
themselves from the omnipotent control of the
jailers, while simultaneously reproaching them
morally."[6]

Abstracting from the comments about the nature of
the jailors and the motivation of the prisoners, this
quote points to some of the important issues with respect to prisoners maintaining their own identity and
retaining some control over their own lives as well as
maintaining a separateness from the system that has imprisoned them and given them a label which they reject.
But again this quotation points out that the primary
intent of the hunger striker is not to die, but rather
to achieve these important psychological and, indeed,
physical realities not necessarily or exclusively for
his or her own self but rather on behalf of himself or
herself as well as their co-prisoners and the cause for
which they were imprisoned.

A second problem with respect to the hunger strikes
comes out from the philosophy of non-violence. Clearly,
the IRA does not embrace the philosophy of non-violence
in any way shape or form. Yet it is important to recall
that in the classical tradition of non-violent protest
the intent of the protester is neither to humble nor
embarrass morally the oppressor. Rather, the one engaged
in non-violent protest attempts to absorb what is perceived to be the evil in a situation and to expose,
through one's own bodily participation, the evil nature
of the situation. Thus the intent of a non-violent protest is to convert the oppressor, not to embarrass or
destroy the oppressor. This is clearly not the case with
hunger strikes. In some ways it is easy to argue that the
purpose of the hunger strike is precisely to embarrass the

British and to shame them into granting the IRA its demands. It may be just as important for the IRA to bring the British to their knees as it would be for them to achieve their change from criminal to political prisoner status or to achieve a united Ireland. There is nothing inherently wrong in trying to use such severely cohersive measures as part of a strategy to achieve one's goals. However, one needs to go beyond reflection on the immediate situation and to recognize that if it should ever be the case that Ireland would be united or, more realistically, if there is to be some sort of political and religious reconciliation in the North, then part of the strategy to achieve that on the part of the Irish should be some willingness to facilitate reconciliation. If the intent of the hunger strike is only to shame and embarrass the British, then a genuine reconciliation will be much more difficult. If the hunger strike were a part of a larger strategy to achieve a change of perspective and an appreciation of the position of the other party, then the hunger strike might be more effective and in fact might appear to be less problematic from a moral point of view to many people.

The hunger strike ended without achieving its major goals, although some concessions were made. Yet the status quo continues: political positions remain hardened, terrorist activity continues on both sides, and the structural problems of Northern Ireland remain unaddressed. Maybe the best the hunger strikes can do is to remind us once again of the seriousness of these issues and of the necessity for both sides to be willing to readdress the issues surrounding the controversies in Ireland and perhaps to effect within their own political parties some means of facilitating a compromise.

FOOTNOTES

1. S. K. Ratcliffe. "Hunger Strikes." Encyclopedia
    of the Social Sciences. New York: The Macmillan
    Company. 1937. Vol. 7. Pp. 552-55.
2. This section summarizes material on the hunger
    strikes reported in Time on 17 August 1981. Pp. 46-
    48.
3. "Ethical Statement: Artificial Feeding of Prisoners."
    British Medical Journal. 6 July 1974. Cf. also
    "The Hunger Striker." Editorial. The Medico-Legal
    Journal. Vol. 42 (1974). P. 59.
4. British Medical Journal, op. cit.
5. For a thorough discussion of paternalism, cf. James
    Childress, Who Should Decide? Paternalism in
    Health Care. New York: Oxford University Press.
    1982. Pp. 102 ff are especially germain to this
    section.
6. Felix Yaroshevsky, M.D., "Self-Mutilation in Soviet
    Prisons." Journal of the Canadian Psychiatric
    Association. Vol. 20. 1975. Pp. 444-45.

NURSING ETHICS

Duties and Dilemmas

The purpose of this paper is to indicate the context of nursing from a personal and professional point of view and then to articulate and discuss three ethical dilemmas in relationship to that context. I do this because my sense is that many of the routine ethical decisions that we make each day of our lives have a significant amount to do with our own personal and professional background as much as they have to do with formal training in ethics or with one's allegiance to a specific religious tradition. I think most of us filter our ethical and religious norms through our personal and professional experiences and make our decisions within that context. With that in mind I would like to spend the remainder of my time discussing the ethical context of nursing, the professional context of nursing and then specific ethical problems that arise within those contexts.

I.   The Ethical Context of the Nurse.

    A.   Personal.

In this section I wish to focus primarily on those experiences that are unique to each individual person and have had a large part to do with who we are in terms of both our personality in the sense of our character as well as the instincts or feelings we have about different issues and the kind of orientation that we have to different problems.

    1.   Family background.

Each one of us comes from a family. Because of the many and varied ways in which this can happen, each of us has unique, special, and significant experiences of and about our family.

Membership in the family gives an individual
the basic affective tone for his or her life, provides a
structure in which an individual can go through the developmental stages of maturity, and helps to mediate values to
the individual as he or she develops. No two families
do any of these things in the same way and each of us has
a different orientation to value issues because of the way
that they were dealt with in our family. The family provides each of us with the base line from which development
in other areas occurs. For better or worse we are in
many ways a specification of who our family is. We can
at a later date reject the values of our family, we can
reject what was done to us by our family and we can also
accept and affirm what was given to us by our family.
But no matter what we do, the experiences that we had
with our family gave us a basic orientation towards
value issues through mediating values to us and through
articulating to us a sense of what kinds of issues,
values and feelings were important. This provides a
significant background in terms of how we perceive
ethical problems.

2.   Religious background

Many people have received religious training
as part of their background. I am talking about religious
training beyond the sense of the religion communicated to
us by our families through participation in worship services,
prayer experiences with the family, as well as the kind of
sense that our family gave us about the mystery expressed
in religion. Many of us have had formal academic training
in religion as well as formal indoctrination into a religion. I am not using indoctrination in a pejorative sense.
By it I simply mean that individuals brought up in a religious tradition are presented with the basic truths of

that religion as well as the moral code that goes with
it before that perspective can be viewed from what I would
consider an academic or formal perspective in which one
examines values, the structure, and the significance of
the content of religion. One of the problems that I
think happens often enough with religion is that our formal academic training in religion stops or at least is
not continued in an appropriate fashion as we begin critical developmental stages from a psychological perspective. Many individuals, then, continue to carry
around with them the images and impressions of religion
which they received through a religious education program
as a child and early adolescent but which they have never
been able to integrate into adult experiences by using
the formal operational modes of reasoning that we use
as we come through adolescence into adulthood. Thus
many individuals have an inherent conflict between the
childhood or adolescent religious ideas that they have
and the adult evaluation of them. Also I think it's
fair to say that within Catholicism in particular, as
well as in many other religions, there has been a
phenomenal liberalization process occurring and many
people simply do not understand what is going on because the leadership has either not been successful in
articulating to the laity what is occurring or because
of resistance to the educational process itself by
leadership and laity alike. This also causes a significant amount of tension and ambiguity. For example,
dissent is now a frequent experience within Catholicism
whereas before it was simply inconceivable that individuals would disagree with their parish priest, much less
the Pope. Our personal religious experiences, education,
and evaluation of those experiences play a tremendous
role in our making ethical decisions. Many will simply

say that because a religion teaches a particular doctrine, that issue is closed to all further discussion. Others will appreciate the significance of the value that the religion is articulating and will attempt to integrate it into contemporary experiences. Still others will reject the religious value out of hand because they do not perceive its meaning or relevance for a contemporary framework. But no matter how each of us personally appreciates religion we have been significantly influenced by having been brought up in a religious environment, by receiving religious indoctrination, and by participating actively in religion. One does not let go of those experiences easily and they are continually present as we select, evaluate, and resolve particular ethical dilemmas.

3.   Personal experiences

In addition to the experience of coming from a family and having a particular religious training each one of us has unique experiences that influence what we see, and what meaning and/or significance we attach to what we see. I am not thinking primarily of experiences that are traumatic although those certainly color what we see. What I am think of primarily is everything that has shaped how we experience a value. Many of these experiences will deal with the sense of appropriateness that we feel when we do something that we consider both correct and fitting to the particular situation at hand. It will also have to do with experiences that we have of doing what we felt was fitting but in reflection realizing that our solution or reaction was not quite appropriate to the particular problem or situation. As we go through life, we accumulate such experiences and these shape how our character is formed, the kind of priorities that we establish in our own life, as well as help shape how we deal with future events.

Thus our personal experiences form another filter through which we see and perceive what is going on around us. Such personal experiences have helped us become liberal or conservative, more open or more closed to new experiences, or more open or more closed to the needs of others. All this influences the context in which values are perceived or ethical decisions are made. They provide in many ways the base line from which all other analysis proceeds.

Thus our family, religious and personal experiences help shape and orientate us to what is of value and the kinds of ethical decisions that we make. Without wishing to belabor what I think is fairly obvious, I think it is still necessary to state these perspectives in a fairly clear way to indicate the basis from which we all began and to indicate the uniqueness of that basis which can give rise to not only our own personal way of seeing a problem but also can go a long way to help us understand why some people do not perceive why other people have problems and vice versa.

B.   Professional

Another significant context is that of the professional training of the nurse. He or she like other professionals undergoes a specialized training and this influences how problems are perceived.   As a professional, a nurse is also governed by a code and I would like to indicate some elements of that as a way of suggesting how ethical dilemmas can be perceived and how one might go about thinking them through.

1.   Training

One of the things that all professionals undergo is a training program which teaches them the particular knowledge that is needed to carry out their specialization. Such training is in part what distinguishes a professional from a lay person and gives the professional

the status and skills necessary to perform at that particular level of expertise. There are several critical
things that I think are important to remember in thinking
about the training that a professional has. First of all
by its very nature the training gives a professional a
jargon and skills that are not readily understood by the
lay person. Thus professionals develop a variety of
acronyms and shorthand ways of discussing problems that
help them communicate efficiently with each other but
makes what they are saying unintelligible to the outsider,
no matter how well-informed that person might be in other
areas. Also when a professional does something, the
assumption is that the professional knows how to do it,
will be competent at doing it, and understands what is
being done. Thus one of the traps that a professional
can fall into is to feel that because he or she understands what is going on everyone else does too. Such
is not always the case and one of the problems that a
professional must deal with is to make sure that what
is being done is made intelligible to the person to whom
it is done. Language and skills separate the professional
from the lay person but they do not of necessity need to
be an insurmountable barrier. They can be if the language
and skills are not explained in a way that makes them
intelligible to the lay person. If they are explained,
the lay person can become more of a partner in undergoing the procedure and this level of understanding and
cooperation may make the entire procedure much easier
and, possibly, safer.

        The second critical dimension of professional
training is that professionals are trained to act. They
are taught a skill and they are taught how to do the
skill well so that a service might be provided. Most
professionals have invested a significant amount of

personal effort and time in learning how to perform the
skills that they have. Nothing, I think, can be more
frustrating to a professional than to learn that someone
wants to reject their particular skill. Such a rejection
is seldom personal but I suspect it would be very difficult for a professional not to take it on a personal
level. It is also difficult, once one has been trained
actively to intervene, to think about the possibility of
not intervening. This, I think, is one of the most difficult things any professional has to think about - not
intervening when every instinct and skill as well as the
whole burden of training and professional socialization
says to intervene. Nonetheless, I think some of the very
critical ethical decisions that health care professionals
need to deal with have to do with not intervening either
because the patient or family has asked that no intervention be made or when the professional him or herself
suspects that there may be a good reason not to intervene.
Such a tension though sets up an incredible dilemma for
the professional and can occasionally be extremely difficult for the professional to resolve.

    2.   Code of Ethics

    One element of the professional-client rela-
tionship is the standards to which the professional is
bound in providing services to the client. Such
standards are generally specified in a code of ethics
which most professional societies now have. Such is
also the case for the American Nursing Association which
has a code of ethics which specifies how a nurse is to
conduct her or himself in providing services to the
client. Such a code, as all codes do, reflects certain
beliefs and values about individuals, nursing as a
profession, health and social values. It is assumed
that the professional will conduct her or his activities
in compliance with these standards which I take to mean

assumes that the member of that association has read, understood, and affirmed these values. Thus, for a code of ethics of a professional society to be effective, its standards must be understood, affirmed, and then practiced by the individual members.

I think it is also important to note that in a code of ethics for a professional society many of the principles have to do with the professional-profession relationship and the steps that a particular profession must take to insure the integrity of the profession and the quality of the relationship between individual persons and society. Such an orientation is extremely helpful because if the members of the profession do not help defend its integrity, it is unlikely that anyone else will; or if things become so bad, society at large will provide such a regulation and this typically has not served the best interest of the profession. Other areas of the code have to do with the professional maintaining an appropriate level of competence as a professional. This is also an important area because these principles are directed to the particular service that the professional provides to a client and if this service is not performed at an appropriate professional level, then individuals can be harmed. Thus, it is important for a professional to take steps to see that he or she maintains an appropriate level of training and that the profession helps insist upon this and provide opportunities to maintain such a level.

Professional codes are also important in terms of how they specify a professional is to help identify and safeguard the interests of the client. The code of ethics of the American Nurses Association is very helpful in this by specifying that services are to be provided with respect for human dignity and the

uniqueness of each client, that the nurses are to safeguard a client's right to privacy through practicing
confidentiality, that a client must be protected from
incompetent, unethical, or illegal practices of any
individuals, and that the nurse is to seek consultation
at appropriate times. Such an orientation towards the
client helps the professional identify their interests
and provides a way to protect them. When a nurse attends
to these particular issues specified by the code, as well
as many others not specified by the code, she or he is
attending to very basic value issues and is establishing
a context in which ethical decisions can be made more
easily when such a situation may present itself. Thus,
on a very pragmatic level, fidelity to the code of
ethics provides another base line by which a nurse
can attend to value and ethical issues within professional practice. Attending to the code provides a way
of helping to see the client in a different framework
so that the interests of the client can be identified
and acted upon.

    C.   Civic

    In addition to being a person and a professional,
a nurse like everyone else, is also a member of society
and as a member of society incurs a variety of obligations. I would like to indicate a couple of these
dimensions and talk about some of the ways which they
can influence one's own personhood as well as one's
professional orientation.

    1.   Obligations Arising from Citizenship

    A nurse, like other members of society, in-
curs obligations arising from that membership. As such,
she or he is responsible for observing the laws of a
particular nation or state and is responsible for
participating in the political process by which such
laws are developed. Thus, nurses must be like other

citizens with respect to practicing civil values and
virtues such as patriotism, appropriate loyalty to civil
leaders, and obedience to the laws of the state.

A nurse may also incur specific obligations
with respect to the law because of her or his participation in a health care setting. A nurse, for example,
must be aware of laws surrounding problems such as child
abuse, the reporting of gunshot wounds, reporting of
venereal diseases, as well as her or his obligation to
report any other problems that may constitute a hazard
to the public health. The nurse, as any other health
care professional, must be aware of special laws that
are relevant to his or her profession and then carry them
out conscientiously. Such carrying out of the law is
basically an exercise of citizenship and constitutes an
expected duty of the members of a particular society.
The nurse, as any other citizen, is expected to exercise
fidelity to the law here, and especially fidelity when
the law involves the matter of health care.

2.   Voluntary Associations

Additionally, the nurse may also be a member
of any number of voluntary associations. This would
range from her or his membership in a nursing organization, a sorority or fraternity, a religious organization, a political party, or some other privately
organized association. What is critical about membership in these associations is that they provide a specific orientation and context to the person as he or
she carries out the routine duties of his or her life. Such
an organization can encourage or at least contribute to
the enhancement of different kinds of values. Membership in a political party, for example, helps promote
the virtue of patriotism, as well as helps the individual participate actively in exercising the obligations

of citizenship. Membership in a religious organization
may foster the development of specific religious virtues or values as a particular way in which the professional can exercise her or his duties. A religious
organization may also help a person practice the corporal
or spiritual works of mercy and may well indeed provide
the motivation that a professional needs to carry out
the duties of that profession.

In any event, the voluntary associations that
we belong to carry us beyond the particular profession
of which we are a member, widen our vision, and help
us attend to value issues that are a routine part of
our day as we exercise professional responsibilities.
Membership in such voluntary associations can help us
become better professionals by making us more sensitive
to the value issues inherent in our personal and social
relationships and by widening our vision so that we can
see things from a perspective that is broader than a
professional.

II. The Professional Context of Nursing

In this section, I would like to focus on three
particular relationships that I think are significant
in defining the context in which nursing is practiced
and therefore have implications for the articulation
and resolution of ethical dilemmas in the practice of
nursing. These three relationships are: male-female
relations, physician-nurse relations, and nurse-patient
relations. Again, without belaboring the obvious, I
hope to lift up specific issues that I think are of
importance to provide a basis for you to think about
some of the routine problems that are present in the
daily practice of nursing.

A.   Male-Female Relations

    1.   Sexual Stereotyping

One of the traditional thematic problems in the relationship between males and females has been the presence of stereotypes of both male and female behavior. Such stereotyping sets up a variety of uncritical assumptions based on prejudice, fears, and what are alleged to be socially desirable and appropriate ways of acting. While one can suggest that such stereotyping has eased relationships by at least making behavior predictable and by givine one a fairly clear role model to follow, it can also be easily and convincingly argued that such stereotyping has also caused a great deal of pain, suffering, and anguish. Problems come, for example, when individuals perceive that the behavior required by the stereotype is neither desirable nor appropriate. Also problems arise when people perceive that the stereotype leads to a genuine stunting of the personality and implicitly closes off a number of personal or career possibilities for a particular individual. Stereotyping may also lead an individual to develop forms of behavior with which he or she may be extremely uncomfortable.

One problem that can arise in the context of nursing is the degree to which the professional role of the nurse is related to dominant cultural sexual stereotypes. The individual in training may perceive the conflict between what the nurse is required to do as a professional and what one's sexual stereotype assumes what that individual may or may not do or what they may or may not be capable of doing. Thus, the professional role of a nurse may suggest that the individual exhibit high degrees of independent judgement. The sexual stereotype may suggest that the individual is not

capable of such independent action. Again, the professional
role of a nurse may suggest that the individual be willing to
enter into personal relationships and exhibit high degrees of
nurturing behavior. Again, the sexual stereotype may suggest
that the individual in question either cannot or should not
exhibit such behaviors. Sexual stereotyping in relation to
the development of a professional can cause serious personal
conflicts which can get translated into a lowering of the
effectiveness of the individual in question. This in itself
is an ethical problem in terms of the training of a professional and such personal conflicts can also translate into
very practical problems on a hospital ward because an
individual may feel that he or she ought not to step out of
the sexual stereotype in which he or she perceives him or
herself to act as the professional that they are trained to
be. Such a conflict can thus cause harm in terms of how a
patient is treated.

    2.   Autonomy and Assertiveness

    One of the specific problems that I think is
causing a great deal of conflict between males and females
is the development among women of a strong sense of
autonomy and assertiveness. I think this is to a large
degree a function of both the women's movement as well as
the fact of women succeeding in areas in which they had
not been allowed to participate before. Women in particular
are perceiving themselves as autonomous individuals, as
having the right to decide on a career and personal plans,
and then to act on these. Women are today less likely
to accept decisions made on their behalf by others than
before. With this is a growing sense that women need to
assert themselves in terms of relationships and in terms
of career development. Such assertiveness, which is
simply speaking up on one's own behalf and in one's
own interest, has, I think, caused a fair amount

of friction between men and women, primarily because it
is a way of breaking out of stereotypic behavior that is
either assumed or expected.

Most men, I think, have trouble dealing with
a strong woman. First, simply because they are not used
to doing that and second, it breaks the usual pattern of
behavior that men have come to expect. Fortunately,
many women are demanding to be taken seriously and assert-
ing themselves so that their needs, concerns, and interests
must be taken into account. I think that we are in for
a rather lengthy and serious transition period in which
men must learn how to deal with the new assertiveness of
women. I think this must be done so that women can begin to assume their rightful and co-equal role in decision
making and so that they can make their own appropriate
decisions about themselves and their careers.

Again, a variety of ethical problems surround the whole issue of autonomy and assertiveness,
both from a personal and structural level. If a person
is not allowed to develop and become autonomous, she or
he will be immature; and a system which encourages such
immaturity through the denial of autonomy to a person
based on stereotypes is an unethical system. Also, if
an individual is simply unreceptive to or will not listen
to an individual who is speaking up on behalf of his or
herself, communications will certainly be inhibited and
critical information about a third party may not be heard
because of an unwillingness to accept another person as
having valid information because such an image does not
fit one's sexual stereotype. Again, my primary point is
that in the context of male and female relationships,
sexual stereotyping and the breaking out of stereotypes
through assertive behavior can cause both personal and
structural ethical dilemmas in terms of how professionals
interact and the consequences of such interactions for
patient care.

B.   Physician-Nurse Relations

1.   Training

The training of nurses and physicians differs in a variety of ways ranging from length of time of education to the theoretical and experiential components of their educations. Each, in his or her training program, develops the specific kinds of necessary expertise, has relevant experiences that teach them to see problems from a variety of perspectives, as well as the opportunity to be in a variety of decision making situations. By their training, physicians and nurses tend to look at the same phenomenon from different points of view and to react to it differently. Such differences in professionalization make it imperative from an ethical point of view that physicians and nurses make sure they are talking about the same phenomenon on the same level and from the same point of view. Differences in training can also lead to differences in knowledge and this can cause conflict also in terms of how one understands a particular problem and how one sees a particular prognosis. Again, such conflict can have an impact on patient care, and physicians and nurses must be attentive to the ethical dilemmas that come from a different factual analysis of a particular situation. My point is that one's training leads one to see certain things from certain perspectives and the kind of training that one has both limits as well as expands one's horizon and that as one is focusing in on a problem, one needs to be aware of the implications that this has for patient care.

2.   Experience

One of the other areas in which there is a possibility of conflict or at least tension between nurses and physicians concerns the different kinds of experiences each one has had with respect to both certain

techniques and the course of various illnesses. Such
a tension becomes immediately apparent in a teaching
hospital in which, in almost all instances, the staff nurses
have had much more experience than the physicians who are
in training. This can range from such a simple thing as
skill in taking a blood sample and escalating all the way
to being able to understand, monitor, and evaluate data
from the various machines that are used in intensive care
units. Nurses simply have to do more things more often
than most physicians do, and because of this, they have
greater skills and facilities in doing such things.
However, conflicts can arise, and such expertise and
experience may not always be welcomed because of its
implications for diminished status on the part of the
physician.

Also nurses spend more time with patients
than physicians do and, as a consequence, they know
much more about a patient at any given moment than a
physician typically does. They also have much more
practical experience in terms of how people progress
through various diseases. They generally have a better
sense of how people respond to various medications and
what complications they should be aware of. This is
not to suggest that physicians are ignorant, unpro-
fessional or incompetent. It is simply a statement of
what I take to be reality; nurses are on duty with a
given set of patients for at least eight hours while a
physician may not be directly in charge of any particular patient for any significant length of time during
any particular day. The familiarity with both patients
and the course of various diseases gives the nurse an
incredible amount of practical experience that can make
her or him much more valuable in terms of being able
to provide critical medical information about a particular patient as well as having a greater degree of

knowledge about a particular patient.

This knowledge based on experience can be the source of tension between physicians and nurses. The nurse's knowledge is also theoretical, but it also contains a great degree of practical experience based on observation and prolonged care of patients. A physician's knowledge is also theoretical; it may be more in depth because of the physician's own training and involvement in patient care. In a particular situation, however, the experience of a physician and a nurse about a particular patient may differ significantly and may lead to tensions in the relationship. The perspective from which one views the patient is extremely important, and when a nurse reports about a patient based on her or his prolonged observation of the patient, such information should be attended to carefully because it reflects the nurse's perception and professional evaluation of the situation. Such an evaluation, even though it may be primarily experiential, is extremely significant and will play a large role in determining what is appropriate patient care. This is a unique contribution that a nurse can make, and he or she must be willing to provide that information and to press for its inclusion in the evaluation of the patient, especially when this information is seen as critical.

3. Team Loyalty

One important feature that helps any organization run smoothly is the concept of team loyalty or team harmony. This occurs when all members of a particular group have reached a consensus or harmony on a particular problem or issue and then each seek in their own ways to reach the objective that has been commonly agreed upon. The commonality of the perception of the problem and acceptance of a resolution of it are

significant factors in achieving successfully the goal
as well as insuring that that goal is reached harmoniously.
Such a situation is also important in the care of a
patient in which all members of the health care team need
to combine their efforts and contribute according to
their particular background to the total well-being of the
patient.

It can often happen, and seems to be happening much more frequently, that such team loyalty understood in this traditional sense is not present. Such
disharmony can arise, for example, from different perceptions of the patient and the relationship of those interests to what is in the patient's best medical interest.
It may be the case that a particular decision by the
attending physician may be in the patient's best medical
interest but may not be perceived by the patient to be
in his or her overall best interests. The patient, for
example, may not wish to undergo heart surgery because
he or she does not feel the benefits are worth the risks,
the expense, or the necessary period of convalescence.
Such a refusal of treatment by a patient may be understood more readily by some members of a health care team
than others. If this occurs and different individuals
take the side of the patient and others take the side of
the physician, team loyalty and harmony soon can disin-
tegrate. Also it may be the case that some members of
a health care team may feel comfortable in discussing
personal matters with patients and may also be comfortable with being a patient advocate, at least in an infor-
al situation. Again this perspective may inject a note
of disharmony in the team because of the different
evaluation of a situation that can come from this different perspective.

Also, it may be the case that a member of a
health care team simply disagrees with either what a
physician is doing, how the physician is doing it, and
the implications of what is proposed to be done for the
patient. This kind of a situation, which I think occurs
often enough, can pose serious personal and professional
problems for the health care team. On the one hand,
there are professional problems in terms of whose responsibility it is to make an appropriate diagnosis and
propose a treatment regimen. That needs to be counter-
balanced with the experience of other members of the
health care team in terms of their understanding of how
such a particular treatment may eventually turn out.
Other problems can arise because it is usually the responsibility of the nursing staff to administer the
medications or at least to certify that the patient has
taken them. A nurse's disagreement with a particular
medication, the way it is administered, or discomfort
with having to help the patient learn to take the medication can cause a significant degree of discomfort among
the staff, and this can have an obvious impact on the
status of the patient.

Nonetheless, it seems to me that it is
appropriate and necessary for different members of the
health care team to articulate problems that they have
even though such articulation may weaken the traditional
team loyalty. I will develop this point more specifically at a later point in the paper. Here, however, I
simply wish to note that calls for team loyalty can
cover substantive problems that need discussion and
resolution. Thus, while each member of a health care
team should recognize that team loyalty and team harmony
are important, they should also remember that this concept
is not the most critical one in terms of exercising one's
personal and professional responsibility towards the
patient.

C.   Nurse-Patient Relations

1.   Care

One of the traditional responsibilities of a
nurse has been to provide direct and personal care to a
patient. I think this is an extremely important responsibility of the nurse especially in light of the contemporary situation in medicine which is relying to larger
and larger degrees on technology in the diagnosis and
treatment of diseases. A not untypical situation is one
in which a patient is surrounded by a variety of machines
whose purpose is either poorly or not at all understood
and in which the patient can be quite uncomfortable and
frequently bewildered. Here the personal and direct care
of that individual by a nurse can serve as a way of
establishing some degree of security within a patient.
Nursing care can provide the necessary reassuring human
touch and can help the patient establish contact with a
world that is familiar and attentive to the needs of the
patient. Such caring does not, I think, have to be that
elaborate. I think, though, that it has to be present
and that it has to be more than attention that is primarily
professional in a narrow sense and only secondarily
personal. By this I do not mean that a nurse must become deeply and intensely involved in each and every
patient. I do think though that a nurse can become
involved with a patient in a caring way so that the
patient can benefit from this distinctly personal touch
in an unfamiliar, if not impersonal, situation. Such
authentic nurturing of the patient by the nurse is beneficial psychologically and physically and is probably one
of the most significant contributions that a nurse can
make to the overall health care of a patient.

2. Loyalty

Another dimension of the nurse-patient relationship that I think is important is the quality of
loyalty to the patient. I think this should characterize
everything that the nurse does. The responsibility for
the care of the patient is placed primarily, but obviously
not exclusively, in the hands of the nurse, and it seems
to me that as a consequence of that responsibility the
nurse must give high priority to being loyal to the
patient, the patient's needs, and the patient's interests.
This means that the nurse should evaluate what she or
he does first of all from the point of view of the patient
and secondarily from other points of view such as schedul-
ing or hospital routine. What I am suggesting is that
the patient is more important than the administrative
structure of the hospital, the routine of the hospital,
or even at times the personal convenience of the staff
of the hospital. Since the nurse is the one who has the
primary responsibility for the routine care of a patient,
the nurse is the one who must establish patient loyalty
as the priority. Such loyalty to the patient will insure
that the patient is treated in a manner befitting his or
her dignity as a human being and in such a way that his
or her health care needs will be attended to in a responsible fashion.

What I am not suggesting in this is that one
should surrender to patient whims, demands, or routine
complaints about the problems that are endemic to every
hospital. Such a suggestion would be both irresponsible
as well as dramatically impractical. What I am suggesting
though is that nurses especially should remember that
their primary loyalty is to the patient and not to a
schedule. Obviously there is a reason why a schedule
and a routine have been developed, but it seems to me

that it is also obvious that a patient's needs can
supersede the reasoning behind a schedule. In those
cases I think it is imperative that the nurse remember
that her or his loyalty is primarily to the patient and
to respond accordingly.

Again, such loyalty to the patient on the part
of the nurse will be of dramatic help to the patient in
recovering. It is another way in which a nurse can affirm the dignity and worth of a patient and make that
patient feel more comfortable in an alien environment.
Such loyalty to a patient is readily perceived by a
patient and is another way in which the patient can
identify a human contact in a strange environment.
Such contact is of significant benefit to the patients
in their long term recovery.

3.   Personal Integrity

Another dimension that is important in the
nurse-patient relationship is the personal integrity of
the nurse. Such integrity has very practical implications
that will show up and be further discussed in a later
section of the paper, but here I simply wish to indicate
that one significant dimension of the relationship is
the fidelity that the nurse maintains to her or his
personal values. One of the easy habits that we fall
into is that of compromising our beliefs and values.
This happens because we perceive that occasionally a
strong stand may be very difficult, counter productive,
or simply not worth the momentary bother. Thus, we find
it quite easy to compromise our beliefs because of the
difficulty of defending them.

However, once again in the nursing context,
fidelity to one's values and beliefs has a significant
impact upon the quality of care that a patient can
receive. If one's personal and professional value system

demands a high degree of loyalty to the patient, then
one must defend the integrity of that stand even though
it may be difficult to do so. If one's values and beliefs demand that one not work in a particular service
or perform particular actions, one must have the courage
of one's convictions and steadfastly refuse compromise.
One must be willing to exert a high degree of personal
autonomy and assertiveness in dealing with others, and
this is not always easy, as we know. Pressures to be
loyal to the team or appeals to greater degrees of knowledge, experience, and expertise or professionalization
make it increasingly more and more difficult to maintain
integrity to one's own belief system. Nonetheless, such
personal integrity and a willingness to stand firm in
one's significant convictions may be the last line of
defense for a patient as well as for one's own sense of
self worth. Taking a stand that is controversial, unpopular, and which causes significant social disturbances
has never been easy, nor is it something that is particularly appealing. Nonetheless, it is one of the most
significant ethical actions one can perform and has the
highest pay-off in terms of the quality of care that is
provided in a health care facility. One's own sense of
personal integrity will help insure high standards of care
and the articulation of appropriate priorities in evaluating patient needs and concerns. Such integrity, I
suggest, is the best safeguard for the quality of the
relationship that exists between patients and nurses.
And because of that it may well be the most significant
ethical quality necessary in a professional.

In these two sections on the ethical context of the nurse and the professional context of the
nurse, I have described some of the routine situations
that I think nurses can experience during their lives

and their careers. None of these things that I have
described strikes me as being exceptional or in
any way unusual. I think one of the problems with many
of these situations that I have described is their very
routineness. We assume that because they happen often
and we have a comfortable way of dealing with them that
the issues presented are not critical. It seems to me
that many of the value dimensions of these situations
that I have described, especially relating to problems
of sexual stereotyping, autonomy, team loyalty, and of
values associated with caring, being loyal to the patient
and personal integrity, have a significant amount to do
with ethical decision making in the practice of nursing.
I think we do not always attend to these garden variety
types of ethical dimensions of nursing because they are
so close to us and because, as I suggested, we have in
some way resolved them. Yet I think it is important in
a context such as this to step back from these situations
to look at our personal, professional, and civic responsibilities and experiences to examine how they influence and shape our perception of a situation. The
same is true in the three elements of the professional
context of nursing that I mentioned. How men and women
typically relate, and how nurses and patients relate
tell a great deal about how an ethical problem will be
perceived, evaluated, and resolved.

Having set out these two dimensions as a
general framework in which ethical problems are perceived
and discussed, I would now like to turn my attention to
some specific ethical dilemmas that I think are important
in nursing.

III.   Specific Ethical Dilemmas

    A.   Obedience to Authority

    In traditional Roman Catholic moral theology the virtue of obedience is ranked quite highly. In fact, occasionally one has the impression that obedience is the only critical virtue. There is a long tradition in Roman Catholic moral theology, as well as in society in general, that we are to obey orders of legitimate authority without questioning them. The assumption is that the one in authority is acting in the best interests of all concerned, may know more about a particular situation than other people, or simply that what is requested is more convenient. When such a framework is combined with a religious perception of authority which relates obedience to human authorities to doing the will of God in a particular situation, the tendency is to accept what the authority says without either challenging it or evaluating it. Such an attitude was reinforced by the presumption that if one followed the legitimate commands of authority, one could not be held personally responsible for any harms that occurred, at least from a moral point of view. The excuse of "I was just following orders." has as long a history in moral theology as it does in politics and the military.

    Such an orientation to authority and obedience has undergone a significant amount of criticism from both a secular and religious point of view in the last few decades. Such criticism has served, I think, as a needed correction to the overemphasis on obedience and authority that has been present especially within Roman Catholic theology.

Obedience to a legitimate authority is an extremely
important value. Obedience is also an extremely important
virtue. I do not in any way wish to reject obedience or
the legitimacy of a person in authority requesting a person to do something. I do think it is important to note,
though, that obedience is neither the most important virtue nor the only virtue. An uncritical single-minded
focusing on obedience can lead to disastrous results because one will tend to exclude material and perspectives
that may be extremely important and which the one person
in authority may not see. Also I think it is important
to recall that in the last few years in Roman Catholic
moral theology there has been a great deal of creative
and helpful work in the area of understanding conscience.
Some of this work has reinforced the traditional perspective on the primacy of the conscience of the individual while other work has focused on the necessity of
forming one's conscience and accepting the responsibility
of evaluating personally a particular situation from an
ethical point of view. Such developments in moral
theology on conscience do not weaken authority or reject obedience. What they do is suggest that respect
for authority and responsiveness to the legitimate commands of authority must be responsible.

In talking about obedience to authority I think we
need to emphasize one's personal responsibility for
evaluating what we are asked to do. The important point
I wish to make here is that from an ethical point of view
it is just as important to justify what we do as it is
to justify what we will not do. From this perspective
obeying the legitimate command of another person needs
as much ethical justification as a decision not to obey
a command, one needs to evaluate how what one is asked
to do squares with one's own value system and with one's

professional perspective. Our obedience should be critical and thoughtful. The fact that we have been commanded
to do something does not in and of itself justify doing
it. I would argue that any action that is commanded needs
to be evaluated, not because one suspects either the
authority who gives the command or the legitimacy of the
authority but simply to insure, as a type of second review,
that what is requested or commanded is in fact morally
appropriate. This is a way of having an individual per-
sonalize and accept full responsibility for what he or
she does. I do not think it is enough from an ethical
point of view to do something simply because authority
commands it. I think that we need to take a second step
and personally acknowledge the appropriateness of that
request with respect to our own standards and our own
professional code of ethics.

Such a perspective may serve to complicate relationships among members of a health care team. This
orientation may cause particular tension between physicians and nurses or between nurses and members of the
hospital administration. A smoothly running operation
is something that is very desirable to administrators
and members of a health care team, and when individuals
begin questioning what is done, the efficiency of the
operation can be disturbed and for some people that is
quite problematic. Nonetheless, I think we have to
recognize that moral integrity is more important than
either efficiency or obedience. I do not think that on
a routine or day-to-day basis, the perspective I suggest of justifying what we are asked to do, as well as
the obvious position of needing to justify what we will
not do, will cause much of a problem. Most things that
we are asked to do are in fact quite appropriate and in
harmony with our personal and professional status. What

I am suggesting primarily is that we acknowledge our
responsibility personally to think about what we are
asked to do and appropriate that decision into our own
selves. I am also suggesting that when an occasional
doubt about the validity or the appropriateness of a
particular request appears to be questionable or
problematic to us, we cannot simply resolve that doubt
by an automatic appeal to either authority or obedience.
Such doubt ought to be resolved before we act upon the
request. And, finally, I suggest that in the extreme
instance when we are not able to justify what is requested of us, we have no choice but to refuse to perform the action.

    B.   Informed Consent

    Informed consent is, I think, the key ethical
concept in medical ethics or bioethics. It addresses
the quality of the relationship between the patient and
the health care provided. It provides the basis for the
discussion of the treatment modalities that are available, as well as the risks and benefits associated with
each one. This allows the individual to evaluate their
impact upon his or her lifestyle and value system. Informed consent also allows the patient and health care
provider an opportunity to discuss their personal and
professional value systems and evaluate what kind of
impact they may have on decisions that need to be made.

    In providing a patient with the opportunity to
give informed consent to a particular treatment or procedure, two ethical values are protected: the autonomy
of the patient and respect for persons. Autonomy is
basically a form of personal liberty of action through
which the individual determines his or her courses of
action in accordance with a plan chosen by him or herself. That is, autonomy involves the dual elements of

deliberating over a variety of plans of action and
selecting one of them and the ability to act in accordance with one's choices. One element without the other
does not make for an autonomous action. Autonomy is an
extremely important value in western civilization and has
always had a special significance within North American
culture. Autonomy allows individuals to exercise self-
determination, allows them to be the master of their
fate, as well as to choose values that appear to be most
appropriate to them. Autonomy is basically the ability
of a person to be his or her own self.

The value of respect for persons means that individuals should not be treated as simply a means but
should be respected as a legitimate end themselves.
Another way to state this is that treating persons with
respect means that we do not manipulate an individual to
achieve our goals. When we treat an individual with
respect we recognize that they are not at our disposal,
that I cannot do something to someone simply because I
want to or because I have certain skills. Respect for
a person means that we accept the otherness of an individual as a center of values. Such an affirmation of
respect affirms the value of another person simply - and
profoundly - as a person and affirms the bodily and
spiritual integrity of that person.

Providing a patient with the opportunity to provide informed consent to a procedure is a way of recognizing the patient as a person and as a way of both protecting and allowing a person to exercise autonomy. If
a patient is not provided with that opportunity, the
patient is relegated to the role of an object whose values
and wishes are not seen as having any significance and is
basically put at the disposal of other individuals.

One of the very critical roles that a nurse can play
is to insure that a patient has had the opportunity to
discuss as completely as the patient wants all of the
implications of the diagnosis and prognosis of a particular illness, as well as the range of treatment modalities available and the implications for his or her lifestyle. I am not arguing that the nurse is the appropriate
or only one to negotiate consent with the patient. I
think this is primarily the task of the physician, but
I think that a nurse can be very helpfully involved in
this by being willing to discuss questions that the
patient has or by informing the physician that a patient
does not seem to understand a particular point that was
discussed. Again, I think the nurse is a logical person
to think of when one raises this issue because the time
that a nurse spends with a person and the awareness that
a nurse can develop of the particular needs or concerns
of a particular patient. By assisting a patient in learning about his or her illness and what kinds of implications
this illness has for one's lifestyle, a nurse can show a
significant amount of respect for persons, as well as
respecting their own autonomy. A nurse may well indeed
have established the rapport with the patient that is
necessary for a patient to open up and begin to talk
about real concerns that may not be discussed with a
physician. Again, the nurse can be very helpful here
in responding to these concerns of the patient directly
through conversations with the patient and indirectly by
reporting these concerns to the physician.

    C.   Truth Telling

On the one hand, telling the truth is a fairly
simple matter: we tell the truth. On the other hand,
how do we tell the truth, how much of the truth do we
tell, and to whom should the truth be told. The problem

of truth telling is reflected in Disraeli's comment that
a gentleman is one who knows when to speak the truth and
when not to.

Such a comment implies that truth telling is dis-
cretionary, that decisions about when to tell or when not
to tell the truth are unilateral and that the rights, needs,
and desires of other persons do not need to be necessarily
taken fully into account. That is, many discussions of
truth telling begin with the assumption that the one in
possession of the truth or knowledge is the primary if
not sole arbiter of what to tell. Such an assumption can
be grounded in the traditional physician ethic of do no
harm or based on assumptions that individuals do not want
to know the truth, that they could not understand it anyway, or more commonly, that they could not deal with it
even if they are told.

I suggest that one's primary obligation lies with
the truth. This is because truth, in general, represents
a reasonably accurate statement of the way things
are, because it affirms the integrity of the relationship
between individuals, and because an individual is entitled to information about his or herself that another
has. There are also some pragmatic reasons for telling
the truth: the person whom we deceive may discover the
truth, and our relationship may be harmed; we may not
remember what we told someone and one lie will lead to
another and eventually into an untenable situation; our
lying may cause people to do or omit things they may have
otherwise done or omitted had they known the truth. In
summary, I think one does not need to justify telling the
truth. One does sense the need to justify telling a lie.
Such a sense argues for at least a prima facie obligation
to tell the truth based on the respect we owe other

persons as autonomous individuals, the respect we owe
other persons as persons, and on the need for trusting
social relationships.

The working situation of a nurse can occasionally
put her or him in an uncomfortable position between the
patient and the physician or between the patient and
family and physician. The nurse generally is in full
possession of all significant medical information about
a particular patient. The nurse knows the diagnosis and
the prognosis and, in general, what the implications
probably are for this particular patient. The physician
is also in the position of possessing relevant knowledge
about a particular patient. The problem is, does the
patient or the patient's family have this knowledge? I
hope it is safe to say that we have passed beyond the time
in which a patient was told absolutely nothing about
his or her condition, including such minor facts as what
one's temperature was. On the other hand, it is not
always apparent that the patient is in possession of the
same knowledge that a nurse or a physician has.

Problems can arise when a patient has not been
informed of something by a physician as should have been
the case, and the nurse is then asked to provide this information. The tension in such a situation is heightened
when the nurse has either been told or has had suggested
to her that the physician is not quite ready to tell the
patient what the problem is. Part of the motivation for
this may be to avoid putting extra stress on a patient at
a critical moment during the course of an illness. It
may be felt that a patient is not in the proper frame of
mind to understand or evaluate the diagnosis, or people
may feel that the individual simply does not want to know.
What happens then when a nurse is asked rather directly
by a patient to provide information that the patient

clearly does not have and more than likely is entitled
to have regardless of whether people think that he or she
should have it' or not?

It is important to realize that one can handle this
situation without lying. A first appropriate response
would be for the nurse to determine factually what the
patient has or has not been told and what the patient
knows or does not know about his or her situation. Such
a response by a nurse does not require any lying whatsoever. Second, the nurse, on the basis of this information
tells the patient or family that he or she will speak to
the attending physician so that such information can be
provided. Third, if the attending physician is either
unwilling or feels it is inappropriate to communicate
such information to the patient or family, the nurse can
speak to her or his supervisor so that the patient can
receive the information that he or she is entitled to.
In this situation, the nurse has not yet told anything to
the patient, but is taking appropriate steps to have that
information provided primarily by people whose obligation
it is to provide that information. When all else fails,
the nurse may appropriately feel that it is her responsibility to provide that information to the patient. I see
nothing wrong with this. The patient is entitled to the
information, and no one else is willing to give it to
the patient. It is important to realize that when a
nurse does that, she or he is stepping into a more advocacy role in terms of the patient, but I think that
is one of the important dimensions of the role of a
nurse in that kind of situation. Again, I think the
first response to a situation like this is to ascertain
what the situation is, to seek to have those people
whose responsibility it is to provide that information

provide it, and if that does not work, and the nurse is
again asked what the situation is, I think it is appropriate
for her or him to provide that information.

Thus, the nurse can quite properly fulfill her or
his obligation to the truth by first seeking to have
appropriate information provided by those whose obligation it is to provide that information, and second, by
assuming an advocacy position on behalf of the patient
and to provide the information to which the patient is
entitled. In this context, however, I do think it is
important for the nurse to ascertain as best as possible
what the facts of the situation are and then to take
appropriate action in the light of those facts. Occasionally there may be an appropriate reason for why the
patient has not been informed at a particular time.
What the nurse can do in that situation is to follow the
case through to make sure that the patient has received
appropriate information when the particular reason for
not providing the information no longer applies. Again
this is a simple   but profound way in which the nurse
can affirm her or his obligations to the truth.

IV.   Conclusions

In this paper I have tried to suggest that the way
in which we see a problem has been shaped by our own
personal life experiences and our professional training.
Each one of us has had unique experiences in one's life
that lead one to see or not see certain problems. Each
one of us has had experiences which make us open or
closed to particular values and each one of us has had
experiences during our professionalization which has made
us responsive or not responsive to particular issues.
I think it is very important to realize and remember that
the context in which we make an ethical decision is
equally as important as the decision that is made. Many

of the dilemmas that each one of us faces on a routine
basis in our lives with respect to ethical decision making
has to do with how different people perceive value issues
about the same situation. I wish to be clear that I am
not arguing for a bankrupt situation ethics or a cultural
relativism. What I am suggesting is that even though
many of us may affirm the same or similar values, we
nonetheless can appreciate them in a different way because
of our life situation and our professional training.
While two people in a discussion may be talking about and
even affirming the same virtue or value, they may perceive
it from slightly different viewpoints which leads them to
draw different conclusions. Thus, for example, in the
nursing context two nurses may both hold the value of the
sanctity of life as a significant value. One nurse,
however, may see that value as leading him or her to do
everything that is possible to preserve the life of a
patient, including the prolonged use of heroic means.
The other nurse may see that value as leading her or him
to terminating extraordinary means when it is apparent
that such means are useless in prolonging the patient's
life even though they may maintain the status quo. Both
begin with the same value but each of them has had particular experiences and training that has led them to
different applications of the value. One of the most
helpful things   each one of us can do in discussions about ethical decisions is to make sure that we
are discussing the same value or principle and that we
share or do not share the common sense of what it means,
as well as trying to understand the varying kinds of
conclusions that may be drawn from that value in a
particular situation.

The major thematic context that I see as problematic in discussions of bioethical issues in general is the constant ambiguity of the situation in which ethical decisions must be made. In the three examples that I provided at the end of my paper - obedience to authority, informed consent, and truth telling - there are so many possible variations of the contexts in which those values occur and the ways in which one may appropriately respond in fidelity to one's values. What I think is most important is the recognition of the fact that there are ambiguities, tensions, and genuinely painful dilemmas in ethical decision making in the context of nursing and medicine. This is not to say that decisions cannot be made or should not be made. I wish to affirm that there are, unfortunately, no clear answers even though we might be quite clear about our values and our standards. In some issues the dilemma may be quite easily resolved but on the other hand there may be a myriad of circumstances which do not admit an easy resolution and a very painful process of negotiation, dialogue and soul searching must occur before we arrive at our decision. What I think is critical and what may be the signal that the most profound ethical reasoning is going on, is the fact that people are troubled about making a particular decision. Such a situation is usually a clue to me that there is the recognition of a value issue at stake and that a person is really struggling with how to find an appropriate and proper resolution for the topic. As long as such a situation continues to be present, I do not become worried about the state of the ethical practice of nursing or medicine. When people sense that there are no problems about decisions or no issues to be debated, I become a little worried and feel that the ethical tone of decision making may be slipping a little.

One of the major difficulties that I see in introducing discussions of ethics into nursing practice and medicine is that I am asking you to complicate your lives when they are already complicated enough. I am asking you to be open to the problems of people in a way that would challenge their value system, as well as test your own value system. I am asking you to be sensitive to the differences of ethics and values which occasionally lead to quite severe tensions between people as individuals with differing backgrounds and perceptions go about attempting to resolve very difficult problems. I would like to bring to you a word of consolation that ethical decision making is easy and that the ethical decisions that you will be making in your practice of nursing will become less complex. I cannot do that and also would argue that those who say that such decision making is easy are leading you astray. However, I can leave you with the word of consolation that if you conduct your professional activities in a highly ethical manner and leave yourself open to the tensions, anxieties, and difficulties of practicing your profession at the highest possible level, I think that you will also experience the joy that comes from the satisfaction of having functioned as an integrated and whole human being and will also have the pleasure of knowing that you have served your patients with the highest personal and professional standards of which you are capable.

Also by the Edwin Mellen Press...

The Emergence of Roman Catholic Medical Ethics in North America: An Historical-Methodological-Bibliographical Study
David Kelly
ISBN 0-88946-887-X   535 pages

The Voice of Illness: A Study in Therapy and Prophecy
Aarne Siirala
ISBN 0-88946-995-4   224 pages

Abortion: An Annotated Indexed Bibliography
Maureen Muldoon
ISBN 0-88946-972-5   200 pages

The Emergence of Roman Catholic Medical Ethics in North America. By
   DAVID F. KELLY. Lewiston, New York: The Edwin Mellen Press, 1979.
   xi + 520 pp.

Given the need for restoring something of the wisdom of natural law ethics
in the face of biomedical prospects for radically altering the meaning of being
human, Professor Kelly offers a timely historical, methodological, and
bibliographical survey of the rich legacy of North American Catholic medical
moral literature. Protestant ethicists may wince in embarrassment. Long
before the contemporary interest in the impact of biomedicine upon human
values, Catholic ethicists, building on traditions of pastoral medicine and
moral theology, applied moral reasoning to the daily procedures of professional medicine. David Kelly, associate professor of moral theology at Saint
Bernard's Seminary, Rochester, New York, has written an informative and
extremely useful account of developments in two periods: (1) 1900–1940,
dominated by an emphasis upon precisely defined physical criteria within
the rubrics of natural law theology, and (2) 1940–1960, when Catholic
medical ethics, under the influence of Pius XII, shifted toward eccelesiastical
positivism. Kelly does well to point out that no sufficient explanation was
given as to why the teaching authority of the church (metaethical supernatural absolutism) should be necessary for deciding medical moral questions
supposedly open to resolution via the application of right reason according to
natural law positivism and its workhorse, the double effect principle. A final
chapter introduces the post-Vatican II movement toward personalism and
holism, a shift, Kelly asserts, marking the end of "Catholic medical ethics as
in any sense distinct" (p. 403).

The author's penchant for repetitive transitional passages, wearisome for
the cover-to-cover reader, may actually enhance the value of the volume as a
reference work. Individual chapters can be examined with profit, especially
if diligent use is made of the extensive footnotes, fifty-page bibliography, and
analytical index. Alternatively, one might use the index of names to chart the
influence of specific Catholic moralists, such as Edwin Healy, Charles
McFadden, and Gerald Kelly. Akin to Protestant criticism of the ahistorical
nature of traditional Roman Catholic natural theology, one wishes that *The
Emergence of Roman Catholic Medical Ethics in North America* exhibited
stronger historicist assumptions, so that shifts in Catholic medical ethics
might be understood more clearly in the context of changing sociocultural
patterns. Nevertheless, Kelly's excellent and necessary study should be a
basic addition to the libraries of all those interested in the history of medical
ethics.

Syracuse University   MILTON C. SERNETT
Syracuse, New York